FAO Fisheries and Aquaculture Report No. 978　　　　　　　　　　　　　　FIPM/R978(En)

Report of the

JOINT FAO/WHO EXPERT CONSULTATION ON THE RISKS AND
BENEFITS OF FISH CONSUMPTION

Rome, 25–29 January 2010

FOOD AND AGRICULTURE ORGANIZATION OF THE UNITED NATIONS
WORLD HEALTH ORGANIZATION
2011

WHO Library Cataloguing-in-Publication Data

Report of the joint FAO/WHO expert consultation on the risks and benefits of fish consumption, 25–29 January 2010, Rome, Italy.

    1.Food contamination. 2.Fish products - toxicity. 3.Fishes - toxicity. 4.Methylmercury compounds - toxicity. 5.Mercury poisoning. 6.Risk assessment. I.World Health Organization. II.Food and Agriculture Organization of the United Nations.

ISBN (FAO) 978-92-5-106999-8
ISBN (WHO) 978-92-4-156431-1 (NLM classification: WA 703)

© FAO/WHO, 2011

All rights reserved. Reproduction and dissemination of material in this information product for educational or other non-commercial purposes are authorized without any prior written permission from the copyright holders provided the source is fully acknowledged. Reproduction of material in this information product for resale or other commercial purposes is prohibited without written permission of the copyright holders. Applications for such permission should be addressed to

    Chief, Electronic Publishing Policy and Support Branch
    Communication Division
    Food and Agriculture Organization of the United Nations (FAO)
    Viale delle Terme di Caracalla
    00153 Rome, Italy
    E-mail: copyright@fao.org;
    or
    WHO Press
    World Health Organization
    20 Avenue Appia
    1211 Geneva 27, Switzerland
    Fax +41 22 7914806
    Requests for permission to reproduce or translate WHO publications – whether for sale or for noncommercial distribution – should be addressed to WHO Press through the WHO web site (http://www.who.int/about/licensing/copyright_form/en/index.html).

The designations employed and the presentation of material in this information product do not imply the expression of any opinion whatsoever on the part of the Food and Agriculture Organization of the United Nations or of the World Health Organization concerning the legal or development status of any country, territory, city or area or of its authorities, or concerning the delimitation of its frontiers or boundaries. The mention of specific companies or products of manufacturers, whether or not these have been patented, does not imply that these have been endorsed or recommended by the Food and Agriculture Organization of the United Nations or the World Health Organization in preference to others of a similar nature that are not mentioned.

All reasonable precautions have been taken by the Food and Agriculture Organization of the United Nations and the World Health Organization to verify the information contained in this publication. However, the published material is being distributed without warranty of any kind, either expressed or implied. The responsibility for the interpretation and use of the material lies with the reader. In no event shall the Food and Agriculture Organization of the United Nations or the World Health Organization be liable for damages arising from its use.

This report contains the collective views of an international group of experts and does not necessarily represent the decisions or the stated policy of the Food and Agriculture Organization of the United Nations or the World Health Organization.

Printed in Italy.

Recommended citation

FAO/WHO (2011). Report of the Joint FAO/WHO Expert Consultation on the Risks and Benefits of Fish Consumption. Rome, Food and Agriculture Organization of the United Nations; Geneva, World Health Organization, 50 pp.

PREPARATION OF THIS DOCUMENT

The thirty-eighth Session of the Codex Committee on Food Additives and Contaminants requested the Codex Alimentarius Commission, at its twenty-ninth Session in 2006, to seek scientific advice from the Food and Agriculture Organization of the United Nations (FAO) and the World Health Organization (WHO) on the risks and benefits of fish consumption: specifically, a comparison of the health benefits of fish consumption with the health risks associated with the contaminants methylmercury and dioxins (defined here to include polychlorinated dibenzo-*p*-dioxins [PCDDs] and polychlorinated dibenzofurans [PCDFs] as well as dioxin-like polychlorinated biphenyls [PCBs]) that may be present in fish. The Codex Alimentarius Commission request was driven by growing public concern in recent years regarding the presence of chemical contaminants in fish. Over the same period, the multiple nutritional benefits of including fish in the diet have become increasingly clear. FAO and WHO held an Expert Consultation on the Risks and Benefits of Fish Consumption from 25 to 29 January 2010 at FAO headquarters in Rome, Italy. Data on levels of nutrients and specific chemical contaminants (methylmercury and dioxins) in a range of fish species were reviewed, as well as recent scientific literature covering the risks and benefits of fish consumption. The review was used to consider risk-benefit assessments for specific end-points, including for sensitive groups of the population.

ACKNOWLEDGEMENTS

The Food and Agriculture Organization of the United Nations (FAO) and the World Health Organization (WHO) would like to express their appreciation to all those who contributed to this Expert Consultation and the preparation of this report, whether by providing their time and expertise, data and other relevant information or by reviewing and providing comments on the document.

Appreciation is also extended to all those who responded to the call for information that was issued by FAO and WHO and thereby drew our attention to references that were not readily available in the mainstream literature and official documentation.

We are sincerely thankful for the budgetary contributions from the Norwegian Ministry of Fisheries and Coastal Affairs, the Japanese Ministry of Health, Labour and Welfare, the Nordic Council of Ministers and the Food and Drug Administration of the United States of America, which allowed us to organize and carry out the Expert Consultation.

FAO/WHO.
Report of the Joint Expert Consultation on the Risks and Benefits of Fish Consumption. Rome, 25–29 January 2010.
FAO Fishery and Aquaculture Report. No. 978. Rome, FAO. 2011. 50 pp.

ABSTRACT

The Food and Agriculture Organization of the United Nations and the World Health Organization convened a Joint Expert Consultation on the Risks and Benefits of Fish Consumption from 25 to 29 January 2010. The tasks of the Expert Consultation were to review data on levels of nutrients (long-chain omega-3 fatty acids) and specific chemical contaminants (methylmercury and dioxins) in a range of fish species and to compare the health benefits of fish consumption and nutrient intake with the health risks associated with contaminants present in fish. The Expert Consultation drew a number of conclusions regarding the health benefits and health risks associated with fish consumption and recommended a series of steps that Member States should take to better assess and manage the risks and benefits of fish consumption and more effectively communicate these risks and benefits to their citizens. The output of the Expert Consultation is a framework for assessing the net health benefits or risks of fish consumption that will provide guidance to national food safety authorities and the Codex Alimentarius Commission in their work on managing risks, taking into account the existing data on the benefits of eating fish. The Expert Consultation concluded the following:

Consumption of fish provides energy, protein and a range of other important nutrients, including the long-chain n-3 polyunsaturated fatty acids (LCn3PUFAs).

Eating fish is part of the cultural traditions of many peoples. In some populations, fish is a major source of food and essential nutrients.

Among the general adult population, consumption of fish, particularly fatty fish, lowers the risk of mortality from coronary heart disease. There is an absence of probable or convincing evidence of risk of coronary heart disease associated with methylmercury. Potential cancer risks associated with dioxins are well below established coronary heart disease benefits from fish consumption.

When comparing the benefits of LCn3PUFAs with the risks of methylmercury among women of childbearing age, maternal fish consumption lowers the risk of suboptimal neurodevelopment in their offspring compared with the offspring of women not eating fish in most circumstances evaluated.

At levels of maternal exposure to dioxins (from fish and other dietary sources) that do not exceed the provisional tolerable monthly intake (PTMI) of 70 pg/kg body weight established by JECFA (for PCDDs, PCDFs and coplanar PCBs), neurodevelopmental risk for the fetus is negligible. At levels of maternal exposure to dioxins (from fish and other dietary sources) that exceed the PTMI, neurodevelopmental risk for the fetus may no longer be negligible.

Among infants, young children and adolescents, the available data are currently insufficient to derive a quantitative framework of the health risks and health benefits of eating fish. However, healthy dietary patterns that include fish consumption and are established early in life influence dietary habits and health during adult life.

DECLARATION OF INTERESTS

The Secretariat ensured that all experts participating in the Expert Consultation had completed declaration of interest forms. Sixteen out of 17 experts declared no substantial economic interest in the topics discussed. One expert had received research grants from industry, but there was no involvement that was considered to be a potential conflict of interest with the issues to be discussed at the meeting.

FURTHER INFORMATION

For further information, please contact:

Fisheries and Aquaculture Policy and Economics Division
Food and Agriculture Organization of the United Nations
Viale delle Terme di Caracalla, 00153 Rome, Italy
Fax: +39 06 57055188
E-mail: FI-Inquiries@fao.org
Web site: www.fao.org

or

Department of Food Safety and Zoonoses
World Health Organization
20 Avenue Appia
1211 Geneva 27
Switzerland
Fax: +41 22 7914807
E-mail: foodsafety@who.int
Web site: www.who.int/foodsafety

ACRONYMS AND ABBREVIATIONS

ALSPAC	Avon Longitudinal Study of Parents and Children
BENERIS	Benefit–Risk Assessment for Food: An Iterative Value-of-Information Approach
BRAFO	Benefit–Risk Analysis of Foods
CI	confidence interval
DALY	disability-adjusted life year
DHA	docosahexaenoic acid
DPA	docosapentaenoic acid
EFSA	European Food Safety Authority
EPA	eicosapentaenoic acid
FAO	Food and Agriculture Organization of the United Nations
IOM	Institute of Medicine
IQ	intelligence quotient
JECFA	Joint FAO/WHO Expert Committee on Food Additives and Contaminants
LCn3PUFA	long-chain n-3 polyunsaturated fatty acid
PCB	polychlorinated biphenyl
PCDD	polychlorinated dibenzo-*p*-dioxin
PCDF	polychlorinated dibenzofuran
PTMI	provisional tolerable monthly intake
QALIBRA	Quality of Life – Integrated Benefit and Risk Analysis
QALY	quality-adjusted life year
TCDD	2,3,7,8-tetrachlorodiobenzo-*p*-dioxin
TEF	toxic equivalent factor
TEQ	toxic equivalent
USA	United States of America
USEPA	United States Environmental Protection Agency
USFDA	United States Food and Drug Administration
WHO	World Health Organization

CONTENTS

PREPARATION OF THIS DOCUMENT iii
ACKNOWLEDGEMENTS iii
ABSTRACT iv
DECLARATION OF INTERESTS v
FURTHER INFORMATION v
ACRONYMS AND ABBREVIATIONS vi

EXECUTIVE SUMMARY .... **IX**

    Background to the Expert Consultation ix
    Scope ix
    Conclusions x
    Recommendations x

1. INTRODUCTION **1**

    1.1 Background 1
    1.2 Terms of reference of the Expert Consultation 1
    1.3 Scope, objectives and target populations 2
        1.3.1 Scope and objectives 2
        1.3.2 Target populations 2

2. RISK–BENEFIT ASSESSMENT **2**

    2.1 Introduction 2
    2.2 Health outcomes 4
        2.2.1 Identification of suitable data sets 4
        2.2.2 Risks 5
        2.2.3 Benefits 8
    2.3 Existing risk–benefit assessments 9
        2.3.1 BRAFO tiered approach for benefit–risk assessment of foods 9
        2.3.2 BENERIS and QALIBRA 10
        2.3.3 EFSA tiered approach for benefit–risk assessment of foods 11
        2.3.4 Risk–benefit analyses using the DALY approach: method development with acid folic as an example 11
        2.3.5 Risk–benefit analyses of fish consumption using the QALY approach ... 11
        2.3.6 Fish risk–benefit assessment by the Institute of Medicine in the USA .. 12
        2.3.7 Quantitative risk–benefit assessment of fish consumption by the USFDA 12
    2.4 Approach taken by the Expert Consultation 13
        2.4.1 Balancing risks of methylmercury and dioxins with benefits of EPA/DHA: rationale 13

    2.4.2 Analyses used to estimate dose–response 14
        2.4.2.1   Methylmercury and neurodevelopment 14
        2.4.2.2   DHA and neurodevelopment 15
        2.4.2.3   EPA plus DHA and mortality from coronary heart disease 17
        2.4.2.4   Dioxins and mortality 19
  2.5 Data on the composition of fish 21
  2.6 Risk–benefit comparison 24
    2.6.1 Neurodevelopment in newborns and infants 25
    2.6.2 Comparison of the effects of methylmercury and DHA on children's IQ: results and discussion 27
    2.6.3 Mortality from coronary heart disease 28
    2.6.4 Comparison of the effects of DHA and dioxins on coronary heart disease mortality: results and discussion 30

3.   **SUMMARY OF FINDINGS** 31
  3.1 Consumption of fish, LCn3PUFAs, methylmercury and dioxins in women of childbearing age, pregnant women and nursing mothers 31
  3.2 Consumption of fish, LCn3PUFAs, methylmercury and dioxins in the general adult population 32

4.   **RESEARCH PRIORITIES AND DATA GAPS** 33

5.   **CONCLUSIONS AND RECOMMENDATIONS** 33
  5.1 Conclusions 33
  5.2 Recommendations 33

6.   **REFERENCES** 34

APPENDIX A: ARITHMETIC MEAN CONTENT OF TOTAL FAT, EPA PLUS DHA, TOTAL MERCURY AND DIOXINS IN 103 SPECIES OF FISH 45

APPENDIX B: MEETING PARTICIPANTS 49

EXECUTIVE SUMMARY

Background to the Expert Consultation

The thirty-eighth Session of the Codex Committee on Food Additives and Contaminants requested the Codex Alimentarius Commission, at its twenty-ninth Session in 2006, to seek scientific advice from the Food and Agriculture Organization of the United Nations (FAO) and the World Health Organization (WHO) on the risks and benefits of fish consumption: specifically, a comparison of the health benefits of fish consumption with the health risks associated with the contaminants methylmercury and dioxins (defined here to include polychlorinated dibenzo-*p*-dioxins [PCDDs] and polychlorinated dibenzofurans [PCDFs] as well as dioxin-like polychlorinated biphenyls [PCBs]) that may be present in fish. The health risks associated with dietary exposure to these compounds have previously been assessed by the Joint FAO/WHO Expert Committee on Food Additives (JECFA).

The Codex Alimentarius Commission request was driven by growing public concern in recent years regarding the presence of chemical contaminants in fish. Over the same period, the multiple nutritional benefits of including fish in the diet have become increasingly clear.

The evolving science in this field has led to questions about how much fish should be eaten, and by whom, in order to minimize the risks of chemical exposures and maximize the health benefits. National authorities have been faced with the challenge of communicating complicated and nuanced messages to consumers and also with questions on how to regulate maximum levels of these chemical contaminants in fish and other foods.

FAO and WHO held an Expert Consultation on the Risks and Benefits of Fish Consumption from 25 to 29 January 2010 at FAO headquarters in Rome, Italy. Seventeen experts in nutrition, toxicology, epidemiology, dietary exposure and risk–benefit assessment discussed the risks and the benefits of fish consumption. Their task was to review data on levels of nutrients and specific chemical contaminants (methylmercury and dioxins) in a range of fish species, as well as recent scientific literature covering the risks and benefits of fish consumption. The review was used to consider risk–benefit assessments for specific end-points, including for sensitive groups of the population. The output is intended to provide guidance to national food safety authorities and the Codex Alimentarius Commission in their work on managing risks, taking into account the existing data on the benefits of eating fish.

Scope

The purpose of the Expert Consultation was to provide a framework for assessing the net health benefits or risks of fish consumption that would assist governments in preparing advice for their own populations.

The terms "fish" and "seafood", which are used interchangeably in this report are defined as finfish (vertebrates) and shellfish (invertebrates), whether of marine or freshwater origin, farmed or wild. Marine mammals and algae, as well as sustainability issues and environmental impacts, although important, are considered to be outside the scope of the report.

Based on the strength of the evidence, the Expert Consultation examined the benefits of fish consumption for optimal neurodevelopment and prevention of cardiovascular disease. Multiple other possible benefits were reviewed in background papers but were not the focus of the Expert Consultation in its consideration of relative risks and benefits. The Expert Consultation also examined the risks to fish consumers of ingesting methylmercury and dioxins.

The Expert Consultation was also requested to conduct an analysis of these benefits and associated risks and make a series of recommendations for target populations, including fetuses, infants and young children, women of reproductive age and high fish consumers, as well as the general population.

Conclusions

The Expert Consultation concluded the following:

- Consumption of fish provides energy, protein and a range of other important nutrients, including the long-chain n-3 polyunsaturated fatty acids (LCn3PUFAs).
- Eating fish is part of the cultural traditions of many peoples. In some populations, fish is a major source of food and essential nutrients.
- Among the general adult population, consumption of fish, particularly fatty fish, lowers the risk of mortality from coronary heart disease. There is an absence of probable or convincing evidence of risk of coronary heart disease associated with methylmercury. Potential cancer risks associated with dioxins are well below established coronary heart disease benefits from fish consumption.
- When comparing the benefits of LCn3PUFAs with the risks of methylmercury among women of childbearing age, maternal fish consumption lowers the risk of suboptimal neurodevelopment in their offspring compared with the offspring of women not eating fish in most circumstances evaluated.
- At levels of maternal exposure to dioxins (from fish and other dietary sources) that do not exceed the provisional tolerable monthly intake (PTMI) of 70 pg/kg body weight established by JECFA (for PCDDs, PCDFs and coplanar PCBs), neurodevelopmental risk for the fetus is negligible. At levels of maternal exposure to dioxins (from fish and other dietary sources) that exceed the PTMI, neurodevelopmental risk for the fetus may no longer be negligible.
- Among infants, young children and adolescents, the available data are currently insufficient to derive a quantitative framework of the health risks and health benefits of eating fish. However, healthy dietary patterns that include fish consumption and are established early in life influence dietary habits and health during adult life.

Recommendations

To minimize risks in target populations, the Expert Consultation recommended a series of steps that Member States should take to better assess and manage the risks and benefits of fish consumption and more effectively communicate with their citizens:

- Acknowledge fish as an important food source of energy, protein and a range of essential nutrients and fish consumption as part of the cultural traditions of many peoples.
- Emphasize the benefits of fish consumption on reducing mortality from coronary heart disease (and the risks of mortality from coronary heart disease associated with not eating fish) for the general adult population.
- Emphasize the net neurodevelopmental benefits to offspring of women of childbearing age who consume fish, particularly pregnant women and nursing mothers, and the neurodevelopmental risks to offspring of women of childbearing age who do not consume fish.
- Develop, maintain and improve existing databases on specific nutrients and contaminants, particularly methylmercury and dioxins, in fish consumed in their region.
- Develop and evaluate risk management and communication strategies that both minimize risks and maximize benefits from fish consumption.

1. INTRODUCTION

1.1 Background

The thirty-eighth Session of the Codex Committee on Food Additives and Contaminants requested the Codex Alimentarius Commission, at its twenty-ninth Session in 2006, to convene a Joint Food and Agriculture Organization of the United Nations (FAO)/World Health Organization (WHO) Expert Consultation on the health risks associated with the presence of methylmercury and dioxins (defined here to include polychlorinated dibenzo-*p*-dioxins [PCDDs] and polychlorinated dibenzofurans [PCDFs] as well as dioxin-like polychlorinated biphenyls [PCBs]) in fish as well as the health benefits of fish consumption. The health risks of methylmercury and dioxins have previously been assessed by the Joint FAO/WHO Expert Committee on Food Additives (JECFA) (FAO/WHO, 2002, 2004, 2007).

In order to better address the request from the Codex Alimentarius Commission and to develop the terms of reference for an Expert Consultation, FAO/WHO held a small expert group meeting in 2007 to get advice on these issues and the most appropriate way forward. The expert group meeting noted that a large number of national studies and assessments were available and that these could form the basis for further development of assessment models and for the evaluation.

FAO and WHO convened a Joint Expert Consultation in Rome, Italy, on 25–29 January 2010 to assess issues associated with the risks and benefits of fish consumption. In particular, the task was to review data on levels of nutrients and specific chemical contaminants (methylmercury and dioxins) in a range of fish species, as well as recent scientific literature covering the risks and benefits of fish consumption, and to consider risk–benefit assessments for specific end-points, including for sensitive groups of the population.

> **Definitions**
>
> *Dioxins*: Polychlorinated dibenzo-*p*-dioxins (PCDDs), polychlorinated dibenzofurans and dioxin-like polychlorinated biphenyls (PCBs)
>
> *Dioxin-like PCBs:* PCBs that act via the aryl hydrocarbon receptor to elicit a range of toxicological responses similar to those elicited by 2,3,7,8-tetrachlorodibenzo-*p*-dioxin (TCDD)
>
> *Fish*: Finfish (vertebrates) and shellfish (invertebrates), whether of marine or freshwater origin, farmed or wild
>
> *Seafood*: Synonymous with fish

1.2 Terms of reference of the Expert Consultation

The terms of reference of the Expert Consultation included the following:

- Assess the health risks associated with fish consumption, particularly relating to methylmercury and dioxins, based on previous JECFA evaluations and focusing on new/additional information required for risk–benefit assessment.
- Assess the nutritional health benefits associated with fish consumption.
- Review the existing risk–benefit assessments of fish consumption at national/regional levels, and consider the applicability of these methodologies/models at the international level.
- Compare the risks and benefits of fish consumption using such a methodology/model.
- Identify data gaps and limitations to the use of such a methodology/model, if any.
- Explore the areas where further consideration will be required.
- Make recommendations to the Codex Alimentarius Commission and Member States on the best approaches to manage the risks and benefits of fish consumption and to communicate these to consumers.

1.3 Scope, objectives and target populations

1.3.1 Scope and objectives

The purpose of this report is to provide a framework for assessing the net health benefits or risks of fish consumption that will assist authorities in preparing advice for their own populations.

The terms "fish" and "seafood", which are used interchangeably in this report are defined as finfish (vertebrates) and shellfish (invertebrates), whether of marine or freshwater origin, farmed or wild. Marine mammals and algae, as well as sustainability issues and environmental impacts, although important, are considered to be outside the scope of the report.

In the report, the benefits of fish consumption for optimal neurodevelopment and prevention of cardiovascular disease are examined, as well as the risks from consuming fish containing methylmercury and dioxins. The contribution to total dietary exposure to dioxins from sources other than fish is not considered.

The report includes an analysis of the benefits and risks from fish consumption and makes a series of recommendations for the target populations. The report does not include consideration of potential benefits of long-chain n-3 (or omega-3) polyunsaturated fatty acids (LCn3PUFAs) from dietary sources other than fish.

1.3.2 Target populations

The target populations for the purposes of this assessment are:

- fetuses, infants, young children and women of reproductive age;
- general population; and
- high fish consumers.

2. RISK–BENEFIT ASSESSMENT

2.1 Introduction

In recent years, the evolving science and debate concerning the benefits and risks of consuming fish have resulted in confusion as to how much, or even if, fish should be consumed, and by whom. International and national food safety agencies have recognized the need to provide useful, clear and relevant information to populations that are concerned about making the healthiest choices when considering whether or not to eat fish. These populations include women of reproductive age, pregnant or nursing women, breastfed infants and young children.

Fish is an integral component of a balanced diet, providing a healthy source of dietary protein and nutrients such as LCn3PUFAs. There is evidence of beneficial effects of fish consumption on lowering the risk of coronary heart disease and stroke, as well as growth and development; in contrast, fish can also contribute significantly to the dietary exposure to some chemical contaminants under some circumstances.

The health benefits and risks are likely to vary according to the fish species, fish size, and harvesting and cultivation practices, as well as the amount consumed and the way in which it is served. While there are a number of potential contaminants of concern in fish, methylmercury and dioxins are the subjects of this report.

Fish and a variety of other organisms from the aquatic environment have been much appreciated as food by humans over the ages. Scientific research since the 1950s has been directed with increasing emphasis to isolating and identifying the beneficial components of fish, followed by demonstrating their effects on health and quantifying their impact.

There is convincing evidence - from extensive prospective cohort studies and randomized trials in humans, together with supportive retrospective, ecological, metabolic and experimental animal studies - that fish consumption reduces the risk of death from coronary heart disease and that fish consumption by women reduces the risk of suboptimal neurodevelopment in their offspring.

There is also emerging, possible or probable evidence that fish consumption may reduce the risk of multiple other adverse health outcomes, including ischaemic stroke, non-fatal coronary heart disease events, congestive heart failure, atrial fibrillation, cognitive decline, depression, anxiety and inflammatory diseases. There is little doubt that LCn3PUFAs, including eicosapentaenoic acid (EPA) and docosahexaenoic acid (DHA), in fish are key nutrients responsible for at least some of these benefits. However, there has been speculation and some emerging evidence that other, non-n3PUFA compounds in fish may contribute to the documented cardioprotective and neuroprotective effects of moderate fish consumption and that the nutritional impact of fish consumption may be greater than the sum of the health benefits of the individual nutrients consumed separately.

It should also be emphasized that for much of the evidence related to the assessment of these health benefits, the measured exposure of interest was fish consumption, which implicitly quantifies the net overall effect, including both the harm and benefit, of fish consumption.

Additionally, health benefits of fish consumption or dietary intake of LCn3PUFAs are often assessed using imprecise dietary estimates, whereas health risks of contaminants are often assessed using objective biomarkers. Substantially greater misclassification, with resulting underestimation of effects, will occur with the former methods.

Fish consumption leads to clear nutritional benefits. Fish provide high-quality protein, minerals and trace elements, fat-soluble vitamins and essential fatty acids, including LCn3PUFAs. A report on seafood risks and benefits from the Institute of Medicine of the National Academies in the United States of America (USA) concluded that eating a low-fat source of protein such as seafood can confer health benefits on the cardiovascular system and on brain and eye development (Nesheim and Yaktine, 2007). Fish consumption may also pose toxicological risks, including neurodevelopmental delay, in fetuses and young children. Thus, women of childbearing age, pregnant or nursing women, and young children are considered sensitive populations for neurodevelopmental risks from exposure to contaminants in fish. Notably, these same groups are also sensitive populations for neurodevelopmental risks from not consuming fish. Methods for quantifying and communicating potential risks and benefits have generally not been comparable.

Understanding how best to communicate the benefits and risks of fish consumption, both real and perceived, to the consumer is a continuing challenge. A 2004 joint advisory by the United States Environmental Protection Agency (USEPA) and the United States Food and Drug Administration (USFDA) recommended that pregnant or nursing women and women who may become pregnant consume up to 340 g (12 ounces) of fish per week overall, consume up to 170 g (6 ounces) of albacore tuna per week and not consume four specific fish species with high mercury levels (USEPA and USFDA, 2004).

However, judging from a large number of research articles (Kuhnlein, 1995; Egeland and Middaugh, 1997; Wiseman and Gobas, 2002; Knuth et al., 2003; Kuhnlein, 2003; Sidhu, 2003; Wong et al., 2003; Sakamoto et al., 2004; Tuomisto et al., 2004; Arnold et al., 2005; Cohen et al., 2005b; Foran et al., 2005, 2006; Gochfeld and Burger, 2005; Hansen and Gilman, 2005; Verbeke et al., 2005; Hooper et al., 2006; Morrissey, 2006; Mozaffarian and Rimm, 2006; Budtz-Jørgensen et al., 2007; Dickhoff et al., 2007; Nesheim and Yaktine, 2007; Verger et al., 2007, 2008; Guevel et al., 2008; Scherer et al.,

2008; Tsuchiya *et al.*, 2008; Ginsberg and Toal, 2009; Gladyshev *et al.*, 2009) and press reports (Hastings, 2006; Squires, 2006a, b, 2007; Bakalar, 2007), it is unclear whether this advisory or other similar advisories have had the intended effect of minimizing risk in the population or instead have increased risk by causing both sensitive populations and the general population to reduce or avoid fish consumption altogether. Thus, evaluating and communicating the risks and benefits of fish have become contentious issues.

Two separate reviews of the literature in 2006 (Mozaffarian and Rimm, 2006; Wang *et al.*, 2006) concluded that the health benefits of fish consumption outweighed the potential risks in the general population. For women of childbearing age, the benefits of modest intake of fish, excepting a few selected species, also outweighed the risks (Mozaffarian and Rimm, 2006). A report on seafood risks and benefits from the Institute of Medicine came to similar conclusions (Nesheim and Yaktine, 2007), as did a draft report on a quantitative risk–benefit assessment of commercial fish consumption that has been made available by the USFDA (2009) for public comment.

A 2007 paper, based on a longitudinal study in the United Kingdom, suggested that advice to limit seafood consumption could actually be detrimental to health. Risks from the loss of nutrients were estimated to be greater than the risks of harm from exposure to trace contaminants in 340 g of seafood (approximately 3 servings) eaten weekly (Hibbeln *et al.*, 2007). Partly based on those data, the National Healthy Mothers, Healthy Babies Coalition issued a recommendation that pregnant women consume no less than 340 g of seafood per week (National Healthy Mothers, Health Babies Coalition, 2007). These seemingly conflicting recommendations have spurred confusion among consumers (Scott, 2007).

The quantification of health risks and benefits for a specific dietary pattern is also challenging. Toxicological risks and nutritional benefits may not be directly comparable and may change in importance during different life stages. Thus, the challenges are cross-disciplinary, reaching across different branches of science. It is no wonder that the public has difficulty interpreting the issues.

2.2 Health outcomes

2.2.1 *Identification of suitable data sets*

The data sets used for the assessment of health outcomes are set out in background papers[1] prepared for the experts for this Expert Consultation. In addition, the Expert Consultation reviewed a small number of very recent, or as yet unpublished, studies and reviews to inform its assessment of health outcomes. These included the second edition of the World Cancer Research Fund and American Institute for Cancer Research (2007) report entitled *Food, Nutrition, Physical Activity, and the Prevention of Cancer: A Global Perspective* and the report of the FAO/WHO Expert Consultation on Fats and Fatty Acids in Human Nutrition (published by FAO in 2010). To judge the levels and strength of evidence, the Expert Consultation agreed to follow the criteria employed in the report of the FAO/WHO Expert Consultation on Fats and Fatty Acids in Human Nutrition (FAO, 2010), which were a modified version of the criteria used in the World Cancer Research Fund and American Institute for Cancer Research (2007) report: *convincing*, *probable*, *possible* and *insufficient*.

---

[1] The background papers will be made available on the websites of FAO (www.fao.org/fishery/publications/en) and WHO (www.who.int/foodsafety/chem/meetings/jan2010/en/index.html).

2.2.2 Risks

> - There is *convincing* evidence of adverse neurological/neurodevelopmental outcomes in infants and young children associated with methylmercury exposure during fetal development due to maternal fish consumption during pregnancy.
>
> - In addition, there is *possible* evidence for cardiovascular harm and for other adverse effects (e.g. immunological and reproductive effects) associated with methylmercury exposure.
>
> - There is *insufficient* evidence for adverse health effects (e.g. endocrine disruption, immunological and neurodevelopmental effects, cancer) associated with exposure to dioxins from fish consumption. The World Cancer Research Fund and American Institute for Cancer Research (2007) report on diet, nutrition, physical activity and cancer prevention did not identify fish consumption patterns as being associated with any cancers, nor did it address exposure to specific chemical contaminants from fish consumption.

A number of epidemiological studies of neurobehavioural development in children have been conducted in populations consuming fish/seafood. The two largest and most carefully performed longitudinal studies were carried out in the Seychelles islands (Davidson *et al.*, 1998; Myers *et al.*, 2003) and the Faroe Islands (Grandjean *et al.*, 1997).

In the Faroe Islands, a data set of more than 1 000 singleton births was assembled, and children were followed for up to 14 years to evaluate exposure parameters and a series of physiological end-points based on a detailed neurobehavioural examination. At 12 months of age, early milestone development (i.e. sitting, creeping and standing) was associated with higher mercury concentrations in hair (Grandjean, Wheihe, and White, 1995). This study therefore suggests that if exposure to methylmercury from human milk had any adverse effect on milestone development in these infants, the effect was compensated for or overruled by the advantages associated with nursing. At age 7 years, decrements in attention, language, verbal memory and, to a lesser extent, motor speed and visual-spatial function and delays in brainstem auditory-evoked potentials were associated with prenatal methylmercury exposure (previously determined from mercury concentrations in cord blood and maternal hair) (Grandjean *et al.*, 1997). A follow-up of these children at 14 years of age still indicated deficits in motor, attention and verbal tests, delayed brainstem auditory-evoked potentials as well as methylmercury-associated alterations of cardiac autonomic activity (Murata *et al.*, 2004; Debes *et al.*, 2006). It should be noted, however, that the diet in the Faroe Islands includes episodic consumption of marine mammals (pilot whales) as well as fish and that the major exposure to methylmercury has been estimated to come from pilot whales (Weihe, Grandjean and Jørgensen, 2005; Debes *et al.*, 2006).

The Seychelles Child Development Study was designed to study the developmental effects of prenatal methylmercury exposure in a fish-eating population. Two longitudinal birth cohort studies, referred to as the pilot study and the main study, were performed, each including more than 700 mother–child pairs. The pilot study on children aged 5–109 weeks did not find any significant association of mercury levels in maternal hair (median concentration: 6.6 µg/g; range: 0.59–36.4 µg/g) with the overall neurological examination, increased muscle tone or deep tendon reflexes (Myers *et al.*, 1995a, b, c; Davidson *et al.*, 2000). The main study, which had several additional covariates and expanded end-points, did not detect any significant adverse outcome in children regardless of their age at testing (Davidson *et al.*, 1998, 2000, 2006; Myers *et al.*, 2003). Rather, the test performance of both cohorts was even enhanced in some instances. Such positive effects have been hypothesized to derive from the intake of beneficial components of fish, such as LCn3PUFAs (Davidson *et al.*, 2000).

In a third, smaller study in New Zealand, a group of children whose mothers had eaten at least three fish/seafood meals per week during pregnancy was studied (Kjellstrom *et al.*, 1986, 1989). The fish species consumed were mainly shark, with average methylmercury levels above 2 mg/kg and reaching a maximum of 4 mg/kg (Kjellstrom et al., 1986; Clarkson and Magos, 2006). A higher prevalence of abnormal results in the Denver Developmental Screening Test was detected in highly exposed children (i.e. maternal hair mercury concentration > 6 μg/g) at age 4, although significance was dependent on whether the outlier was included (Kjellstrom et al., 1986). At age 6, poorer scores on full-scale intelligence quotient (IQ), language development, and visual-spatial and gross motor skills were associated with maternal hair mercury concentrations in the range of 13–15 μg/g (Kjellstrom et al., 1989; Crump et al., 1998).

Using data from these three studies, conducted in the Faroe Islands, the Seychelles islands and New Zealand, three meta-analyses established a dose–response relationship between maternal methylmercury body burden, expressed as mercury concentrations in maternal hair, and child IQ (Cohen et al., 2005b; Axelrad et al., 2007; USFDA, 2009).

More recently, an ongoing study of a birth cohort in Massachusetts, USA, showed an association of methylmercury exposure with neurodevelopmental effects at lower exposures than in prior studies (Oken et al., 2005, 2008a). In contrast, a new mother–child cohort, recruited in 2000 (Davidson et al., 2008; Strain et al., 2008) from the high fish-eating population of the Seychelles, showed a positive association between maternal serum DHA levels and accumulating neurodevelopmental benefits at 9 and 30 months of age in children from mothers with methylmercury burdens indicated by mercury concentrations in maternal hair up to about 11 μg/g (Lynch et al., 2011).

Some epidemiological studies provide limited evidence of an association between methylmercury body burden, primarily from fish consumption, and cardiovascular disease. A study of 1 833 Finnish men followed prospectively showed a doubling of risk for myocardial infarction in the highest tertile of exposure (hair mercury concentration > 2 μg/g) (Salonen et al., 1995). A follow-up of this population from eastern Finland continued to show a heightened risk of coronary events due to methylmercury exposure, which was able to offset the positive influence of LCn3PUFA intake in fish (Virtanen et al., 2005). A prospective study of 1 014 Finnish men found that those in the highest quintile of methylmercury exposure (hair mercury concentration > 2.81 μg/g) had an accelerated thickening of the carotid artery, an indication of atherosclerosis (Salonen et al., 2000). In the same study, some evidence of increased cardiovascular mortality in men in relation to hair mercury concentration was reported (Salonen et al., 1995; Virtanen et al., 2005). A similar association was noted with either hair or toenail mercury concentration in two other studies (Rissanen et al., 2000; Guallar et al., 2002). In a case–control study spanning eight European countries and Israel, 684 men with myocardial infarction were found to have a significantly higher toenail mercury concentration compared with the 724 matched controls (Guallar et al., 2002).

However, several other studies failed to find an association between mercury body burden and cardiovascular outcomes (Ahlquist et al., 1999; Hallgren et al., 2001; Yoshizawa et al., 2002). A study of 1 462 Swedish women did not find an association between serum mercury level and incidence of stroke, but this study was focused primarily on mercury exposure via amalgam fillings (Ahlquist et al., 1999). In another Swedish study, this time involving 78 men and women with myocardial infarction and 124 controls, mercury concentration in toenails was found to be correlated with myocardial infarction risk (Hallgren et al., 2001). Overall, this study may not have had sufficient power to detect an independent effect of methylmercury on myocardial infarction, especially given the low exposures to methylmercury in this population.

A large prospective study of health professionals in the USA collected toenail mercury data from 33 737 men, 470 of whom had a myocardial infarction during the course of follow-up (Yoshizawa et al., 2002). The overall analysis showed no difference in risk of myocardial infarction across the quintiles of toenail mercury concentration, but there was also no demonstrable benefit from fish ingestion, in contrast to other studies. The majority of subjects were dentists, and they were overrepresented in the highest exposure groups. The authors reported a positive but non-significant association of mercury concentration in toenails with coronary heart disease in a sub-analysis that excluded dentists. Overall, mechanistic evidence and results of experimental animal toxicological, human clinical toxicological and epidemiological studies support the notion that methylmercury might be a risk factor for cardiovascular disease.

A relatively recent study by Valera, Dewailly and Poirier, 2009, found that exposure of Nunavik Inuit adults (Northern Quebec, Canada) to environmental mercury was associated with increased blood pressure and pulse rate. Furthermore, Lim *et al.*, 2010, reported that in a community in the Republic of Korea, low-dose mercury exposure (average mercury concentration in hair: 0.83 µg/g) was associated with altered cardiac autonomic activity, possibly through an action of mercury on parasympathetic functions.

Studies of the effects of methylmercury on the sex ratio of offspring at birth and stillbirth in Minamata City, Japan, in the 1950s and 1960s, including the period when methylmercury pollution was most severe, showed decreases in male births in the overall city population as well as among fishing families (Sakamoto, Nakano and Akagi, 2001; Itai *et al.*, 2004). An increase in the proportion of male stillborn fetuses raises the possibility that an increased susceptibility of male fetuses to death in utero could explain the altered sex ratio.

Inorganic mercury was shown to suppress immune functions and to induce autoimmunity in multiple species (Silbergeld, Silva and Nyland, 2005). Both methylmercury and inorganic mercury were shown to produce an autoimmune response as well as an immunosuppressive effect in several strains of genetically susceptible mice (Haggqvist *et al.*, 2005). However, data on the immune effects of methylmercury in general are scarce, and research is required in this area.

Dioxins can cause a variety of adverse health effects, including cancer and non-cancer health effects on the immune system, reproductive system, nervous system, endocrine system and others. However, most of the evidence has been based on occupational or accidental exposures at high doses and extrapolation from experimental animal studies. Little evidence is available from well-planned cohort studies.

Raaschou-Nielsen *et al.* (2005) conducted the largest prospective study to examine the association between PCBs and organic chlorinated pesticides and breast cancer in postmenopausal women in Denmark; it was the first prospective study to use stored adipose tissue in the exposure assessment. They found no risk patterns or statistically significant results for the sum of PCBs or any of the PCB congeners in relation to either all breast cancers or estrogen receptor positive breast cancers. The final results did not indicate that higher organochlorine body levels increased the risk of breast cancer in postmenopausal women.

The Expert Consultation also reviewed the World Cancer Research Fund and American Institute for Cancer Research (2007) report on diet, nutrition, physical activity and cancer prevention, which examined the relationships between fish consumption and cancers at 13 sites (identified in relation to diet). This report concluded that fish consumption was associated in a protective manner with colorectal and pancreatic cancer (limited suggestive evidence). In addition, nutrients commonly found in fish were identified as protective for some cancer sites: selenium (probable for prostate, limited suggestive for stomach) and vitamin E (limited suggestive for oesophageal). The World Cancer Research Fund and American Institute for Cancer Research (2007) report did not identify fish consumption as being associated with any of the 13 major diet-related cancers assessed in the report. However, a specific fish preparation (Cantonese salted fermented fish) was identified as being convincingly associated with nasopharyngeal cancer. Even though the report addressed dietary exposure alone and did not include or specifically address exposure to contaminants from fish, the Expert Consultation concluded that these results suggest that dioxins in fish are not a significant risk factor for cancer.

Many epidemiological studies have examined the association of gestational and lactational exposure to dioxins and non-dioxin-like PCBs with neurobehavioural development. However, it is not possible to distinguish the contribution specific to dioxins from the overall results; in other words, the relative contribution of non-dioxin-like PCBs cannot be separated from that of dioxin-like PCBs. Nevertheless, experimental animal data, including those from non-human primates, are supportive of the notion that dioxins can cause developmental neurotoxicity.

2.2.3 Benefits

- There is *convincing* evidence of beneficial health outcomes from fish consumption for:
  - reduction in risk of cardiac death; and
  - improved neurodevelopment in infants and young children when fish is consumed by the mother before and during pregnancy.

- Evidence of other health benefits ranges from *probable* (e.g. ischaemic stroke) to *possible* (e.g. mood and depression) to *insufficient* (e.g. cancer).

- The benefits of fish consumption, demonstrated in numerous studies across a wide range of populations, reflect the sum of benefits and risks from all of the constituents in the fish.

- The health attributes of fish are most likely due in large part to LCn3PUFAs. Fish, however, contain other nutrients (e.g. protein, selenium, iodine, vitamin D, choline and taurine) that may also contribute to the health benefits of fish. The health effects of fish consumption may be greater than the sum of its individual constituents. Eating fish is also part of the cultural traditions of many peoples. In some countries, where viable options for substitute foods are extremely limited, fish is the major source of protein and other essential nutrients.

- Based on the observed dose–response relationships and heterogeneity of background diets, it is very unlikely that the benefits of fish are explained to any large extent by the replacement of less "healthy" foods with fish. However, if this were to be the case, it would still represent a causal effect of fish consumption.

- The majority of studies of fish have examined finfish consumption, although many have included shellfish in their consideration of total LCn3PUFA intake.

- Findings from the multiple clinical, metabolic and experimental studies using fish oils are considered to support the benefits of fish consumption.

DHA is preferentially incorporated into the developing brain during the last trimester of pregnancy and the first 2 years after birth, concentrating in brain grey matter and retinal membranes (Martinez, 1992; Lewin *et al.*, 2005). Multiple observational studies have demonstrated independent beneficial associations of DHA levels in maternal blood during pregnancy or in cord blood during delivery or of maternal fish consumption during pregnancy with more optimal neurodevelopmental outcomes in offspring. These neurodevelopmental outcomes include better behavioural attention scores, visual recognition memory and language comprehension in infancy and childhood (Colombo *et al.*, 2004; Daniels *et al.*, 2004; Oken *et al.*, 2005; Hibbeln *et al.*, 2007). These observational findings are consistent with findings of randomized controlled trials of DHA supplementation during nursing. Together, they demonstrate that maternal consumption of LCn3PUFAs (particularly DHA) during pregnancy and nursing improves early brain development in children.

Nineteen prospective cohort studies and five randomized clinical trials together provide strong evidence that consumption of n-3PUFAs from either fish or fish oil supplements lowers the risk of cardiovascular disease, especially death from coronary heart disease and sudden cardiac death (Kromhout *et al.*, 1985; Burr *et al.*, 1989; Dolecek and Granditis, 1991; Fraser *et al.*, 1992; Kromhout, Feskens and Bowles, 1995; Daviglus *et al.*, 1997; Mann *et al.*, 1997; Albert *et al.*, 1998, 2002; GISSI-Prevenzione Investigators [Gruppo Italiano per lo Studio della Sopravvivenza nell'Infarto miocardico], 1999; Oomen *et al.*, 2000; Yuan *et al.*, 2001; Hu, Bronner and Willett, 2002; Burr *et al.*, 2003; Lemaitre *et al.*, 2003; Mozaffarian *et al.*, 2003, 2005; Osler, Andreasen and Hoidrup, 2003; Folsom and Demissie, 2004; Nakamura *et al.*, 2005; Yokoyama *et al.*, 2005). The dose–response relationship between consumption of n-3PUFAs and mortality from coronary heart disease or sudden cardiac death appears non-linear: compared with little or no intake, modest intake (~250–500 mg EPA plus DHA per day) lowers relative risk, and higher intakes do not substantially further lower mortality from coronary heart disease. A pooled analysis of 20 large studies in humans demonstrates this non-linear effect for death from coronary heart disease, with a 36 percent risk reduction up to 250 mg EPA plus DHA per day and then little additional lowering of risk at higher doses (Mozaffarian and Rimm, 2006). Results were very similar when restricted only to prospective cohort studies of seafood consumption in generally healthy (primary prevention) populations (Harris *et al.*, 2009). Thus, overall benefits of fish or fish oil consumption for death from coronary heart disease appear very similar in prospective cohort studies of fish consumption in generally healthy populations (i.e. primary prevention) compared with controlled trials of fish oil in individuals with established heart disease (i.e. secondary prevention). Effects did not appear to vary depending on whether patients were receiving anti-platelet medications, beta-blockers, angiotensin-converting enzyme inhibitors or statins (Marchioli *et al.*, 2007). Population groups included in these cohorts and trials, which included studies in the USA, Europe, Asia and Australia, were varied, suggesting that coronary heart disease benefits are applicable across a wide range of countries and background diets.

2.3   Existing risk–benefit assessments

Several international risk–benefit activities can serve as examples for the kind of framework needed for the quantitative consideration of the risks and benefits of fish consumption.

2.3.1   BRAFO tiered approach for benefit–risk assessment of foods

The Benefit–Risk Analysis of Foods (BRAFO) project developed a tiered approach for performing risk–benefit assessments (Hoekstra *et al.*, 2010). As with all tiered assessment approaches, the aim was to refine the assessment only as far as is necessary to reach a decision, in this case on whether the net health impact of a dietary change is beneficial or adverse. The approach considers a risk–benefit assessment as a comparison of a reference scenario with at least one alternative scenario (e.g. a policy or an intervention). The assessment starts with a pre-assessment and problem formulation stage in which these two scenarios are further developed and the scope of the assessment is set. After that, four tiers follow:

1) In Tier 1, each risk or benefit is assessed independently. These assessments will often use standard screening methods, but it may be worth using more refined methods if this avoids the need to proceed to Tier 2. Tier 1 comprises a separate, but as comprehensive as needed, risk assessment and a separate benefit assessment.
2) In Tier 2, risks and benefits are compared in a qualitative way. At this stage, no common metric is used; however, the assessment of each individual risk or benefit can be quantitative or even probabilistic.
3) In Tier 3, risks and benefits are integrated quantitatively in a common metric by a deterministic approach.
4) In Tier 4, risks and benefits are integrated quantitatively in a common metric by a probabilistic approach.

The steps needed to reach a conclusion in each tier largely follow the steps included in the Codex risk assessment paradigm (FAO/WHO, 2010). However, the first tier is followed by comparison (Tier 2) and integration (Tiers 3 and 4) of the risks and benefits. This approach is shown in Figure 1.

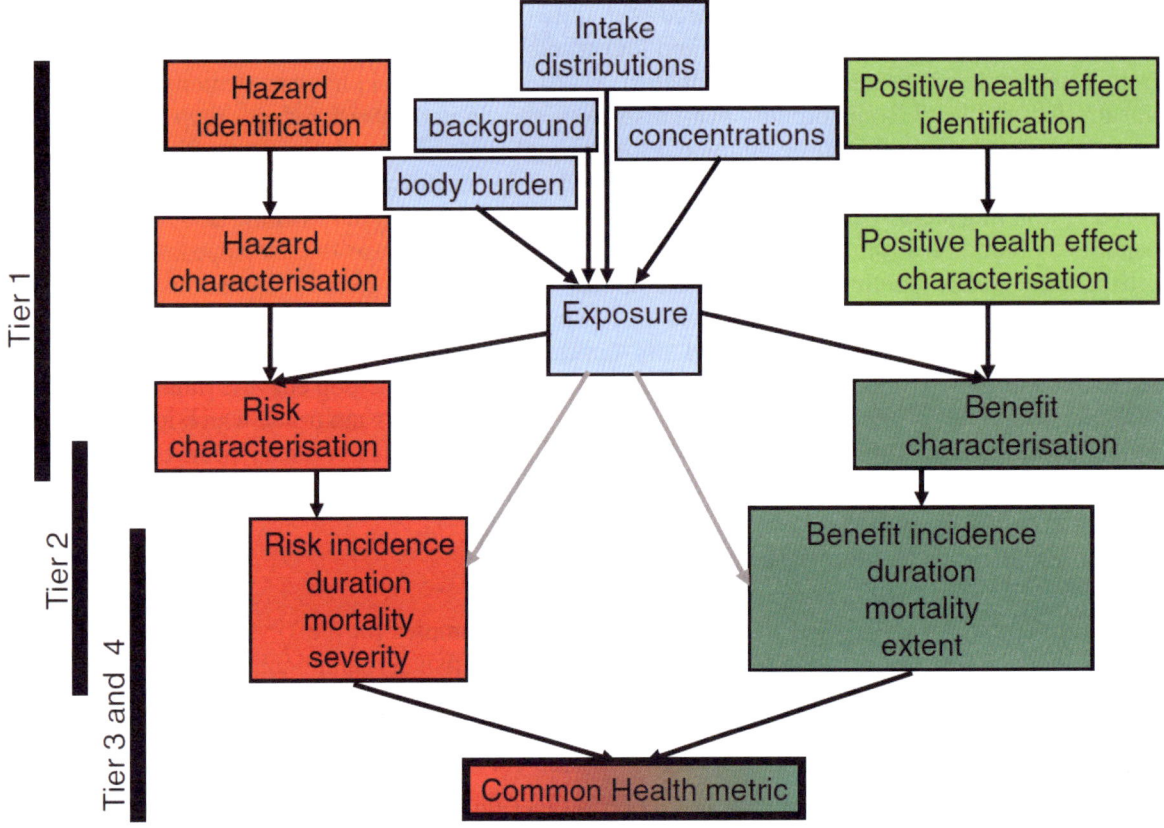

Figure 1. A schematic description of the steps within each BRAFO tier (BRAFO, 2010)

The methodology has been tested with a number of case-studies, including a case-study on fish (Watzl *et al.*, 2011).

2.3.2 BENERIS and QALIBRA

Two other examples of risk–benefit assessment methodology include ongoing studies from the European Union: Benefit–Risk Assessment for Food: An Iterative Value-of-Information Approach (BENERIS) and Quality of Life – Integrated Benefit and Risk Analysis (QALIBRA).

BENERIS aims to advance the science of food risk–benefit analysis for human health (Vartianen *et al.* 2006). The project has a focus on the development of methodological tools that integrate both epidemiological and toxicological data to analyse food risks and benefits. BENERIS allows for the integration of data from food consumption and nutrient intake studies from a number of European countries with chemical contaminant measurements to assess exposure to both contaminants and nutrients in food. More information is available from the BENERIS project web site at www.beneris.eu.

QALIBRA is a related project that has as a goal the development of web-based risk assessment tools that use flexible, modular approaches for integrating exposure estimates and dose–response relationships to evaluate the risks and benefits of foods. The project is coordinated by Matis Ltd – Icelandic Food and Biotech R and D. The tool will assess and also communicate net health impacts resulting from multiple risks and benefits from particular foods, as well as associated uncertainties. QALIBRA also aims to develop web-enabled software that would be available to all stakeholders and includes different components that can be adapted to different user groups, including scaling current national fish risk–benefit assessments to the international level. For more information, the reader should visit the QALIBRA project web site at www.qalibra.eu.

2.3.3 EFSA tiered approach for benefit–risk assessment of foods

The Scientific Committee of the European Food Safety Authority (EFSA) developed guidance for performing risk–benefit assessments of food (EFSA Scientific Committee, 2010). The document focuses on human health risks and human health benefits and does not address cost-effectiveness or other ethical, social or economic considerations.

It is considered as essential that formulation of the problem precedes the risk–benefit assessment. A stepwise or three-tiered approach is recommended for the risk–benefit assessment, with the outcome of each step of the assessment including a narrative of the strengths and weaknesses of the evidence base and its associated uncertainties.

The EFSA opinion is a guidance document similar to the BRAFO methodology. Both methods identify the need for proper problem formulation before the actual assessment is performed, and there is overlap between the tiers/steps.

2.3.4 Risk–benefit analyses using the DALY approach: method development with folic acid as an example

A paper by Hoekstra et al. (2008) describes a method for risk–benefit analyses and uses fortification of bread with folic acid as an example, expanding a method that is already used in risk assessment. Steps include 1) hazard and benefit identification, 2) hazard and benefit characterization through dose-response functions, 3) exposure assessment and 4) risk-benefit characterization through integration of risks and benefits by expressing them in a common metric, such as the disability-adjusted life year (DALY).

2.3.5 Risk–benefit analyses of fish consumption using the QALY approach

Through a case-study of the risks and benefits of fish consumption, Ponce and colleagues (Ponce et al., 2000; Ponce, Wong and Faustman, 2001) explored approaches involving the use of alternative weighting schemes such as quality-adjusted life years (QALYs) to adjust dose–response models. Although this analysis assessed only one risk and one benefit, it demonstrates the utility of the method and its general applicability to other public health decisions. Furthermore, this analysis provides a means to improve upon current health policy analyses conducted on the basis of comparing risks of adverse health impacts. These analyses typically assume that the health end-points for risk are of equivalent detriment or impact, but such a situation is rarely the case, as health impacts differ in terms of both severity and duration.

Using the common metric of QALYs, Cohen et al. (2005a) integrated the results of four studies by an expert panel to assess the aggregate health impact on prenatal cognitive development, mortality from coronary heart disease and stroke resulting from hypothetical shifts in fish consumption. Three scenarios assessed potential population responses to measures such as advisories that encourage women of childbearing age to eat less fish contaminated with mercury. Two other scenarios assess responses to measures such as consumer education that encourages older adults to eat more fish. Specifically, the four quantitative studies, which are described in more detail elsewhere, form the basis of this aggregate impacts paper that assessed the influence of methylmercury exposure on prenatal cognitive development (Cohen, Bellinger and Shaywitz, 2005b), the influence of LCn3PUFA (DHA) intake on prenatal cognitive development (Cohen et al., 2005c), the effects of fish consumption on coronary heart disease mortality (Konig et al., 2005) and the effects of fish consumption on stroke risk (Bouzan et al., 2005).

It should be pointed out that Cohen *et al.* (2005a) assessed the health impacts of only one contaminant (methylmercury only, not dioxins), did not address additional health outcomes (e.g. cancer risk) and did not consider the impact of shifts in diet away from fish (e.g. possible higher cardiovascular disease risk due to higher saturated fat intake). The authors did perform uncertainty analyses using the Monte Carlo method and sensitivity analyses to test various assumptions in their model. Guevel *et al.* (2008) subsequently used a QALY approach to conduct a risk–benefit analysis of high fish consumption in France.

2.3.6 Fish risk–benefit assessment by the Institute of Medicine in the USA

In 2006, as a result of conflicting consumer messages and lack of consensus in the scientific community, the National Oceanic and Atmospheric Administration in the USA commissioned a report by the Institute of Medicine of the National Academies, with support from the USFDA, to evaluate the risks and benefits associated with seafood consumption. The report also sought to make recommendations for consumers in the USA, aiming to create a more comprehensive understanding that would enable consumers to make educated decisions when selecting seafood (Nesheim and Yaktine, 2007).

The Institute of Medicine (IOM) developed a step-by-step decision framework, which evaluated the risks and benefits of seafood consumption based on scientific evidence to examine four population groups: 1) females who are or may become pregnant or who are breastfeeding, 2) children up to 12 years of age, 3) healthy adolescent and adult males and females (who as defined by the IOM report will not become pregnant) and 4) adult males and females who are at risk of coronary heart disease. A decision pathway was then created with this information, highlighting the factors for categorizing consumers in specific target groups that face different benefits and risks and that should receive appropriately tailored advice.

The report acknowledges the complexities involved in consumer decisions and the strong influence that the "information environment" has on these decisions. Consumer seafood choices do not always reflect the new and evolving information being published. For many consumers, seafood selection involves weighing the trade-offs of consumption.

2.3.7 Quantitative risk–benefit assessment of fish consumption by the USFDA

In 2008–2009, the USFDA (2009) undertook an ambitious quantitative risk–benefit assessment of fish consumption that examined both potential for fetal neurodevelopmental effects from methylmercury exposure and coronary heart disease and stroke prevention in the general population. The neurodevelopmental impacts that were examined in this report focused primarily on verbal development.

The USFDA (2009) report contains specific flow diagrams for exposure and dose–response modelling. The flow diagram for exposure modelling is informative, as it shows how specific studies from multiple sources were integrated and, along with accompanying tables, shows specifics about study strengths and limitations. The flow diagram for the dose–response modelling illustrates how each of the knowledge gaps in the dose–response model is addressed in terms of assumptions made and the implications of those assumptions. The USFDA (2009) report contains a very current review of the primary literature that was performed for this very large risk–benefit assessment. It is of particular note, as the utility of the data from each study is reviewed for their applicability to risk–benefit analysis.

2.4 Approach taken by the Expert Consultation

2.4.1 *Balancing risks of methylmercury and dioxins with benefits of EPA/DHA: rationale*

After reviewing the literature, the Expert Consultation decided to compare the effects of 1) prenatal exposure to LCn3PUFAs and methylmercury on child IQ and 2) exposure to LCn3PUFAs and dioxins on mortality. The rationale for this choice is based on the common health end-points and relatively robust evidence to establish dose–response relationships from multiple cohort studies that provide the basis for a quantitative risk–benefit analysis.

The fetus is susceptible to environmental influences. Fish consumption during gestation can provide the fetus with LCn3PUFAs and other nutrients essential for growth and development of the brain. However, fish consumption also exposes the fetus to the neurotoxicant methylmercury. A number of meta-analyses have established linear dose–response relationships between dietary exposure to LCn3PUFAs and methylmercury and child IQ.

Various studies in human populations have examined the association of gestational and/or lactational exposure to dioxins and non-dioxin-like PCBs with neurobehavioural development. These include the Great Lakes cohort (Jacobson and Jacobson, 2003), the Dutch cohort (various studies; see Schantz, Widholm and Rice, 2003 for review) and the Oswego, USA, cohort (Stewart *et al.*, 2008). In the Dutch cohort study, initiated in 1987, it was originally reported that higher levels of PCBs, PCDDs and PCDFs in breast milk (as an exposure index of prenatal and early neonatal exposure) were related to reduced neonatal neurological optimality in infants (Huisman *et al.*, 1995). A follow-up study in the same cohort reported a delay in maturation of at least 1 year in brain areas related to visual-motor and cognitive performance in children with higher prenatal and cumulative lactational dioxin exposure (Leijs *et al.*, 2008). All studies identified neurobehavioural alterations in children examined up to age 8. For example, Stewart *et al.* (2008) identified a 2.9 point decrease in full-scale IQ for every 1 ng/g of PCB exposure (placental levels). Although various populations have been documented to have elevated body burdens of PCBs (e.g. National Health and Nutrition Examination Survey 2001–2002 results: median serum PCB levels in United States residents 20–49 years of age range from 160 to 249 ppb (lipid based); Nichols *et al.*, 2007), the potential quantitative impact of PCB exposure on full IQ development is difficult to define accurately at this time. A problem with all these studies is that the contribution specific to dioxins cannot be delineated from the overall contaminant results; in other words, the relative contribution of non-dioxin-like PCBs cannot be separated from that of dioxin-like PCBs. Nevertheless, experimental animal data, including those from non-human primates, are supportive of the conclusion that dioxins can cause developmental neurotoxicity.

Because of these difficulties, a quantitative evaluation of developmental exposure to dioxins with relation to body burden and IQ was not carried out by the Expert Consultation; however, levels of dioxins in fish should be considered in any risk–benefit analysis done with fatty fish, as dioxin levels in fish and lipid content (including DHA and EPA) show strong correlations. It should also be recognized that for some fish species, depending on the location, total PCBs are significantly and positively correlated to the total toxic equivalent (TEQ) contribution from PCB TEQs (Bhavsar *et al.*, 2007). The **"Toxic Equivalent" (TEQ)** compares the toxicity of the less toxic dioxin and dioxin-like PCB compounds – to the most toxic – TCDD. Each compound is attributed a specific **"Toxic Equivalency Factor" (TEF)**, which indicates the degree of toxicity compared to 2,3,7,8–TCDD, which is given a reference value of 1. The World Health Organization defines the TEQ as the quantified level of each individual congener multiplied by the corresponding TEF. TEQs of each congener are summed to achieve and overall toxic equivalents for a sample (WHO, 1998).

In contrast, the Expert Consultation finds the evidence to be conclusive for decreased mortality from coronary heart disease as a result of dietary exposure to LCn3PUFAs from fish consumption and for the increased risk of mortality due to cancer as a result of exposure to dioxins, albeit at levels resulting from accidental or occupational exposure.

The following section describes the rationale and the quantitative relationships adopted by the Expert Consultation in calculating the effects of methylmercury and LCn3PUFAs on child IQ and the effects of dioxins and LCn3PUFAs on mortality.

2.4.2 Analyses used to estimate dose–response

2.4.2.1 Methylmercury and neurodevelopment

The Expert Consultation considered dose–response models presented in three meta-analyses relating maternal methylmercury body burden, expressed as mercury concentrations in maternal hair, to child IQ. Two of the analyses (Cohen et al., 2005b; Axelrad et al., 2007) were based on the three major cohort studies conducted in the Faroe Islands, New Zealand and the Seychelles. These studies included a battery of tests conducted on children aged 7–9 years. A third analysis (Carrington and Bolger, 2000) utilized pooled data on developmental milestones in children aged 1–3 years from Iraq and the Seychelles.

The analysis developed by Axelrad et al. (2007) for the USEPA developed integrated estimates of IQ from three different prospective epidemiological studies: New Zealand, Seychelles and the Faroe Islands. The estimates from each cohort are presented in Table 1.

Table 1. IQ decrement per microgram per gram of mercury in maternal hair in Axelrad et al. (2007)

Study	Linear slope[a]	Population size[b]	Notes
New Zealand	-0.50 ± 0.027	237	Reported in Table III of Crump et al. (1998); outlier child omitted; rescaled to study population variance
Seychelles	-0.17 ± 0.13	643	Reported in Table 2 of Myers et al. (2003); rescaled to study population variance
Faroe Islands	-0.124 ± 0.057	917	Reported in Axelrad et al. (2007), based on structural equation modelling of three IQ subtests by Budtz-Jørgensen et al. (2005)

[a] Mean ± standard error.
[b] Population size reflects final study group size used for the dose–response evaluation.

Axelrad et al. (2007) used a Bayesian analysis to integrate the results from these three studies, which resulted in an estimate of a single slope of −0.18 (95 percent confidence interval [CI]: −0.38 to −0.01). The Axelrad et al. (2007) analysis is similar to one used in support of a USEPA regulation for mercury in air (USEPA, 2005). The difference is that the previous analysis (Ryan, 2005) used the IQ scales as originally reported, whereas Axelrad et al. (2007) rescaled the results using study population variances.

The analysis conducted by Cohen, Bellinger and Shaywitz (2005b) was presented as part of a larger analysis concerned with the risks and benefits of fish consumption. This analysis integrated results from three different prospective epidemiological studies: New Zealand (Kjellstrom et al., 1989), the Seychelles islands (Myers et al., 2003) and the Faroe Islands (Grandjean et al., 1997). The responses, or end-points, were a wide range of behavioural tests of children aged 7–9 years. Instead of working with raw data, Cohen et al. (2005b) relied on regression analyses conducted by the original authors of the studies. Although the results are not based on a standard IQ test, they were converted to a scale that is comparable to IQ. However, because the regression analysis from the Faroe Islands uses the log of mercury concentration in maternal hair as the dose metric, it was necessary to convert this dose metric by "linearizing" the regression, which involves assuming that the dose–response relationship is linear over a relatively narrow dose range.

In order to facilitate comparison with the New Zealand and Seychelles islands analyses, linear coefficients were developed from the Faroe Islands study using the reported low end of the log (dose)-linear slope. This range was chosen because it most closely matches exposures in the USA, and the resulting slope of −0.7 IQ point per microgram of mercury per gram of maternal hair was used as the principal dose–response model in their cost–benefit analysis (Cohen, Bellinger and Shaywitz, 2005b). However, this slope is based on the use of a log-linear model to extrapolate from Faroe Island exposures to much lower levels of exposure in the USA, where this model yields implausible results: as the mercury dose gets progressively smaller, the IQ decrement approaches infinity. In order to address this problem, Cohen, Bellinger and Shaywitz (2005b) also reported a secondary "sensitivity" analysis where the linear coefficients were taken from the range of exposures that predominated in the Faroe Island cohort, which resulted in an average slope of −0.2.

Carrington and Bolger (2000) developed a dose–response function to represent the relationship between maternal exposure to methylmercury, using hair mercury concentration as a marker for exposure, and the age of onset of walking and talking. This analysis was based on pooled data from the Iraqi mercury poisoning episode in the early 1970s (IPCS, 1990) and milestone data obtained from the prospective epidemiological study in the Seychelles (Myers *et al.*, 1995a, b, c). The resulting functions were approximately linear. When converted to an IQ scale by comparing the milestone decrements to ranges of normal variation, the central estimates of the dose–response functions corresponded to slopes of −0.20 and −0.41 IQ points per microgram of mercury per gram of hair for age of talking and age of walking, respectively.

After reviewing all the evidence presented in the publications, the Expert Consultation decided to use the following linear estimates of the dose–response relationship for the risk–benefit analysis: −0.18 IQ as the central estimate (from the Axelrad *et al.*, 2007 analysis) and −0.7 as the upper limit (from the Cohen, Bellinger and Shaywitz, 2005b analysis).

To convert methylmercury concentrations in fish to mercury concentrations in maternal hair, three assumptions were made: 1) the serving size is 100 g, 2) body weight is 60 kg and 3) the ratio between mercury concentration in hair and daily methylmercury exposure expressed as micrograms per kilogram body weight per day is 9.3. This ratio was calculated based on a one-compartment model previously used by WHO (1976).

2.4.2.2 DHA and neurodevelopment

The Expert Consultation considered dose–response data presented in several studies relating maternal DHA consumption to measures of child neurodevelopment. Generally, different neurodevelopment scales were converted to estimated IQ using z-scores (standard deviations) of distribution, with a one standard deviation difference considered equivalent to 15 IQ points.

Cohen, Bellinger and Shaywitz (2005b) is a meta-analysis of eight randomized controlled trials of DHA supplementation to mothers. Seven of these trials tested DHA supplementation during nursing; only one trial tested DHA supplementation that started during gestation and continued into nursing. The meta-analysis found that for every 100 mg/day of maternal DHA consumption, child IQ increased by 0.13 point (95 percent CI: 0.08–0.18). Multiple different developmental scales were evaluated in these studies, converted to IQ scores using z-scores. Age of evaluation for the children ranged from 6 months to 4 years. The pooled estimate for the benefit of DHA for total IQ was 17 percent lower than the estimate for the benefit of DHA for verbal IQ using one weighting scheme and similar to the original estimate using another weighting scheme.

The Expert Consultation concluded that this meta-analysis of randomized controlled trials provided direct confirmation of a causal benefit of maternal DHA consumption on child IQ, but that the quantitative magnitude of this effect was likely to be underestimated, given that nearly all of these trials evaluated the effects of DHA only during nursing, rather than during both gestation (a critical period of sensitivity for neurodevelopment) and nursing. Thus, this meta-analysis was utilized qualitatively to confirm evidence for the neurodevelopmental benefits of DHA, with the quantitative dose–response relationship derived from prospective cohort studies assessing relationships between maternal DHA consumption during gestation and child IQ, described below. The Expert Consultation further noted that use of prospective cohort studies for defining this quantitative dose–response relationship was also consistent with the methods for determining relationships between maternal methylmercury exposure during gestation and child IQ, described above.

The USFDA (2009) analysis utilized data from the Avon Longitudinal Study of Parents and Children (ALSPAC), a prospective cohort of 7 223 mother–child pairs, to derive a dose–response relationship between maternal fish consumption and child verbal IQ. Because ALSPAC data provided information on fish consumption, average DHA consumption from fish was estimated by the Expert Consultation using fish-specific DHA levels weighted by market share in the USA and using a bootstrapping technique to account for uncertainty. Overall, average fish consumption was estimated to provide a total of 6 mg of EPA plus DPA plus DHA per gram of fish, 5.4 mg of EPA plus DHA per gram of fish and 3.6 mg of DHA per gram of fish. Thus, consuming 27.8 g of fish per day was estimated to provide, on average, 100 mg of DHA. Two different analyses of relationships between fish consumption and child verbal IQ in ALSPAC were considered:

1) Daniels *et al.* (2004) assessed the relationship between maternal fish consumption, evaluated over four categories, and child IQ at 18 months of age. This analysis resulted in a non-linear dose–response relationship, with each gram per day of maternal fish consumption improving child IQ by 0.104 point (95 percent CI: 0.032–0.288) until a fish consumption level of 18.2 g/day (95 percent CI: 8.9–55.9), with no further IQ gain thereafter. These analyses were adjusted for age and infant fish consumption. Based on an average concentration of 3.6 mg of DHA per gram of fish, this corresponds to 2.8 points of verbal IQ gain (95 percent CI: 0.89–8.0) per 100 mg/day DHA intake until a level of 65.5 mg/day DHA (95 percent CI: 32.0–201.2), with no further IQ gain thereafter. Based on this regression, the calculated maximum potential IQ gain would be 1.8 IQ points.

2) Hibbeln *et al.* (2007) assessed the relationship between maternal fish consumption, evaluated over six categories, and child IQ at 8 years of age. The estimates provided by the authors were adjusted for multiple demographic and social covariates. The analysis of the data also produced a non-linear dose–response relationship, with each gram per day of maternal fish consumption improving child IQ by 0.152 point (95 percent CI: 0.104–0.212) until a fish intake level of 30.5 g/day (95 percent CI: 24.7–51.4), with no further IQ gain thereafter. Based on an average of 3.6 mg of DHA per gram of fish, this corresponds to 4.2 points of verbal IQ gain (95 percent CI: 2.9–5.9) per 100 mg/day DHA intake, until a level of 110 mg/day DHA (95 percent CI: 89–185), with no further IQ gain thereafter. Based on this regression, the calculated maximum potential IQ gain would be 4.6 IQ points.

In the ALSPAC study, the actual observed IQ difference between the highest and lowest categories of maternal fish consumption was 5.5 points. Thus, both of these regression analyses appeared to underestimate the maximum potential IQ gain, with the latter analysis being a smaller underestimate.

Oken *et al.* (2008a) assessed the relationship between maternal fish consumption and child IQ at 3 years of age in Project Viva, a prospective cohort of 341 mother–child pairs in the USA. Maternal fish consumption in the second trimester was assessed by a food frequency questionnaire. Child IQ was estimated from the child picture vocabulary test and visual-motor abilities test at 3 years. These analyses were adjusted for multiple covariates and for red blood cell mercury levels. Maternal fish consumption of more than two servings per week, compared with none, was associated with a 0.16 standard deviation greater picture vocabulary test score and a 0.61 standard deviation greater visual-motor abilities test score, or an average (mean) 0.38 standard deviation gain on these two neurodevelopment tests. Based on 15 IQ points per standard deviation, the Expert Consultation estimated a 5.8 IQ point gain across these categories of fish consumption. Assuming median fish consumption of 3 servings per week in the highest category, with an average of 3.6 mg of DHA per gram of fish and an average serving of 100 g, this corresponded to an average of 154 mg of DHA per day in the highest category of fish consumption. Thus, the results of this study correspond to 3.8 points of IQ gain per 100 mg/day maternal DHA intake, with a maximum IQ gain of 5.8 IQ points, based on the actual observed difference between the highest and lowest categories of fish consumption.

The Expert Consultation also considered the analysis of Oken *et al.* (2008b) in the Danish Birth Cohort of 25 336 mother–child pairs. Maternal fish intake was assessed at 25 weeks of pregnancy (second trimester), and child developmental milestones were assessed at 18 months of age and used to create a total development scale. Significant associations were seen in analyses considering the risk of a child being below specific neurodevelopmental cut-off points, but no linear IQ analyses were presented to allow calculation of a dose–response relationship. Thus, these data were viewed as qualitatively supportive but did not contribute to the dose–response estimate.

In summary, based on the available data, together with additional experimental evidence reviewed separately, the Expert Consultation concluded that there was convincing evidence for benefits of maternal DHA consumption during gestation on neurodevelopment in their children. The Expert Consultation further concluded that their differing quantitative analyses from different prospective cohorts, each utilizing different metrics and divergent assumptions, showed consistent dose–response relationships between maternal DHA consumption and child IQ. In particular, the most reliable multivariable-adjusted estimates from two different cohorts, ALSPAC and Project Viva, demonstrated similar IQ gains of 4.2 and 3.8 points per 100 mg of DHA per day, respectively, or an average of 4.0 points IQ gain per 100 mg of DHA per day. The Expert Consultation recognized that this value could be an overestimate of benefit due to residual confounding, but it could also be a substantial underestimate of benefit due to misclassification (error) in the estimations of both maternal DHA consumption and child IQ. In terms of maximum potential benefit, the Expert Consultation concluded that the most conservative approach should not extrapolate expected benefits beyond observed IQ differences (even though such benefits could exist). Thus, the maximum observed IQ gain across categories of fish consumption (5.8 IQ points) was considered to be the maximum potential IQ gain from maternal DHA (from fish) consumption, with no further benefits with increasing consumption thereafter.

However, the Expert Consultation recognized that there are cultures and populations with low or no fish consumption. Specific studies on neurodevelopment of these particular populations, on which strong conclusions could be drawn, have not been performed.

2.4.2.3 EPA plus DHA and mortality from coronary heart disease

The Expert Consultation considered dose–response data presented in several studies relating intake of EPA plus DHA to coronary heart disease mortality. These included prospective cohort studies of fish consumption and coronary heart disease mortality in generally healthy populations (primary prevention) and randomized controlled trials of fish or fish oil consumption in populations with underlying coronary heart disease or mixed populations with and without coronary heart disease (primary and secondary prevention). The general concordance and consistency of the different studies did not provide strong evidence for effect modification by the presence or absence of underlying coronary heart disease, so the entirety of evidence was considered together. Two separate pooled analyses were utilized to derive a dose–response relationship.

Mozaffarian and Rimm (2006) pooled the results of 16 prospective cohort studies and 4 randomized controlled trials that evaluated the effects of EPA plus DHA intake on coronary heart disease mortality. In this analysis, the authors converted fish consumption to intake of EPA plus DHA using study-specific estimates or imputations based on similar populations. Among observational studies, only fully multivariable-adjusted risk estimates were used. The analysis included a total of 326 572 individuals in prospective cohort studies and 35 115 individuals in randomized controlled trials from the USA, Europe and Asia. The pooled risk estimate from these 20 studies demonstrated a highly significant inverse association between EPA plus DHA intake and risk of coronary heart disease mortality, with a non-linear dose–response relationship. For intakes between 0 and 250 mg of EPA plus DHA per day, the risk of coronary heart disease mortality was 36 percent lower (95 percent CI: 20–50 percent), corresponding to 16.3 percent lower risk per each 100 mg/day. At intake levels greater than 250 mg/day, no further decrease in coronary heart disease mortality was seen (0.0 percent lower risk per 100 mg/day; 95 percent CI: −0.9 percent to 0.8 percent). A separate analysis including only the primary prevention prospective cohorts demonstrated very similar results (Harris *et al.*, 2009).

USFDA (2009) utilized 16 cohorts, consisting of the 13 cohorts identified and used in the meta-analysis of He *et al.* (2004a) plus 3 additional studies that met the study criteria and were published afterwards (He *et al.*, 2004b; Cohen, Bellinger and Shaywitz, 2005b; Axelrad *et al.*, 2007). Fish consumption (g/day) was used as the exposure metric. Although the results across studies were not entirely consistent, which suggests the possibility of systematic differences between cohorts, as a whole, the studies indicated a benefit from the consumption of up to 25 g of fish per day, with coronary heart disease mortality decreased by 25.6 percent. Additional fish consumption above 25 g/day appeared to provide little or no additional risk reduction.

In summary, based on the available data, together with additional evidence for the effects of EPA plus DHA and fish consumption on cardiovascular risk factors, the Expert Consultation concluded that there was convincing evidence for the benefits of EPA plus DHA intake on coronary heart disease mortality. The Expert Consultation also concluded that both quantitative analyses provided concordant results, with one analysis evaluating EPA plus DHA intake as the exposure and the other evaluating fish consumption. Thus, the results of the first analysis were considered appropriate for quantifying the coronary heart disease mortality benefits of EPA plus DHA intake, and the results of the second analysis for quantifying the coronary heart disease mortality benefits of fish consumption.

Reduction in coronary heart disease mortality from intake of EPA plus DHA was estimated as follows:

$$\text{Deaths prevented per million people} = \frac{[EPA + DHA] \times 100 \times x/7}{250} \times 0.36 \times D$$

where:

- $[EPA + DHA]$ is the total concentration of EPA plus DHA in fish (mg/g);
- 100 is the estimated fish serving size (g);
- x is the number of servings of fish per week (7 days);
- 0.36 is the proportional reduction in coronary heart disease deaths, with reduction in deaths assumed to be linearly related to DHA intake up to 250 mg/day;
- D is the estimated number of coronary heart disease deaths per million people (1580 deaths per year per million people, calculated over 70 years).

Again, as for the conclusions on neurodevelopment, specific studies of coronary heart disease mortality, on which strong conclusions could be drawn, have not been performed in populations that do not eat fish.

2.4.2.4 Dioxins and mortality

As reported by a WHO Consultation (WHO, 2000), the most informative studies for the evaluation of the carcinogenicity of dioxins are four cohort studies of herbicide producers (one each in the USA and the Netherlands, two in Germany) and one cohort study of residents in a contaminated area in Seveso, Italy. In addition, a multi-country cohort study by IARC (1997) includes three of the four high-exposure cohorts and other industrial cohorts, many of them not reported in separate publications, as well as some professional herbicide applicators.

In most epidemiological studies considered, exposure was to mixtures of PCDDs, including 2,3,7,8 tetrachlorodibenzo-*p*-dioxin (TCDD), as contaminants of phenoxy herbicides and chlorophenols. The cohorts examined in these epidemiological studies do not allow an evaluation of the risk associated with exposure to higher PCDDs separate from exposure to TCDD.

Increased risks for all cancers combined were seen in the occupational cohort studies. The magnitude of the increase was generally low; it was higher in sub-cohorts considered to have the heaviest TCDD exposure. Positive dose–response trends for all cancers combined were present in the largest and most heavily exposed German cohort and in the smaller German cohort where an accident occurred with the release of large amounts of TCDD. Increased risks for all cancers combined were also seen in the longer-duration, longer-latency sub-cohort of the study in the USA and among workers with the heaviest exposure in the Dutch study. These positive trends with increased exposure tend to reinforce the overall positive association between all cancers combined and exposure (Kogevinas, 2000). The large German cohort evaluated dose–response relationships for estimated exposure to both TCDD and PCDDs/PCDFs using international TEQs and identified a positive trend in both analyses. In Seveso, all-cancer mortality did not differ significantly from that expected in any of the contaminated zones, although excess risks were seen for specific cancers. Follow-up for the Seveso cohort was shorter than for the occupational cohorts. In most of these studies, excess risks were observed for soft tissue sarcoma and also for lung cancer, non-Hodgkin lymphoma and digestive tract cancers. Statistically significant excess risks were observed in individual cohorts for a variety of other cancers, including multiple myeloma, oral cavity cancer, kidney cancer, leukaemia and breast cancer in women.

A single study in Seveso (Pesatori *et al.*, 1993) examined cancer in children 0–19 years of age. Excess risks were observed for thyroid cancer and for some neoplasias of the haematopoietic tissue; these results were based on small numbers.

Two studies have evaluated cancer risk among subjects exposed to contaminated rice oil in Japan (*Yusho*) and Taiwan, China (*Yu-Cheng*). The terms *Yusho* and *Yu-cheng* literally mean "oil disease" in Japanese and Chinese respectively. The Japanese oil contained PCBs at concentrations in the order of 1000 mg/kg and PCDFs at concentrations in the order of 5 mg/kg. Estimates of intake are based on a study of 141 cases (Hayabuchi, Yoshimura and Kuratsune, 1979). These patients consumed about 600 ml of oil over about one month and ingested about 600 mg of PCBs and 3.5 mg of PCDFs total. Assuming a body weight of 60 kg, the daily doses were thus 0.33 mg of PCBs per kilogram of body weight per day and 0.002 mg of PCDFs per kilogram of body weight per day. The oil from Taiwan, China, contained about 100 mg of PCBs per kilogram and 0.4 mg of PCDFs per kilogram. Estimates are based on a study of 99 cases. Patients consumed about 1 g of PCBs and 3.8 mg of PCDFs over a period of about 10 months. Daily doses were approximately 0.06 mg PCBs per kilogram of body weight per day and 0.0002 mg PCDFs per kilogram of body weight per day. The contaminated rice oil contained a complex mixture of chlorinated ring compounds, including dioxin-like and non-dioxin-like PCBs, polychlorinated quaterphenyls and polychlorinated terphenyls, as well as the PCDFs. There was an excess liver cancer risk in Japan (odds ratio: 3.1) at 22 years of follow-up, and there was no excess risk in Taiwan, China (odds ratio: 0.8), at 12 years.

In summary, the epidemiological evidence from the most highly TCDD-exposed cohorts studied produces the strongest evidence of increased risks for all cancers combined, along with less strong evidence of increased risks for cancers of particular sites. The relative risk for all cancers combined in the most highly exposed and longer-latency subcohorts is 1.4 (WHO, 2000). While this relative risk is not likely to be explained by confounding, this possibility cannot be excluded. It should be borne in mind that the general population is exposed to 2–3 orders of magnitude lower levels of TCDD and 1–2 orders of magnitude lower levels of PCDDs/PCDFs than those experienced, as an equivalent lifetime dose, in the industrial populations examined or the population at Seveso.

It is important to note that JECFA, in its assessment of dioxins, concluded that there was likely to be a threshold associated with any cancer risk from dioxins and that setting a health-based guidance value based on effects other than cancer – for example, immune suppression and reproductive effects – would also address any carcinogenic risk (FAO/WHO, 2002).

In the worst case, consuming a single fish meal containing dioxins at a concentration of 20 pg/g with the lowest concentration of EPA plus DHA ($\leq$3 mg/g) results in the lowest net benefit for mortality reduction. In general, however, when considering an upper estimate for theoretical increased cancer incidence from dioxins in fish, the defined benefits of fish consumption from reduction of coronary heart disease mortality exceed any hypothetical cancer risk.

The long half-lives of dioxins have several implications for the period of intake that is relevant for risk assessment:

- The concentration of dioxins in the body will increase continually over time as more of the compounds are ingested.

- Because of the long half-lives of these compounds in humans, the intake on a particular day will have a small or even negligible effect on the overall body burden.

- For women of reproductive age, consideration should be given to avoiding continual consumption of fish with high concentrations of dioxins because of transfer in utero and post-parturition (lactation) to the developing human. To minimize risk, chronic consumption patterns should be avoided where the provisional tolerable monthly intake (PTMI) of 70 pg/kg body weight established by JECFA for PCDDs, PCDFs and coplanar PCBs (FAO/WHO, 2002) is being exceeded on a continual basis.

- While recognizing that there are a number of food commodities that can contribute to overall exposure to dioxins, for some populations (i.e. subsistence lifestyle), dioxin exposure from fish consumption may make a significant contribution to overall dietary exposure. In certain cases, the PTMI for dioxins can be exceeded by over 10-fold by consumption of fish with high levels of dioxins (Table 2).

Table 2. Daily dietary exposure to dioxins through consumption of 100 g servings of fish one, two or seven times per week, for an individual with a 60 kg body weight[a]

Servings per week (100 g per serving)	Dioxin concentration (pg/g)	Dietary exposure to dioxins (pg/kg body weight per day)
One serving	0.2	0.05
	2.5	0.60
	6.0	1.43
	20	4.76
Two servings	0.2	0.10
	2.5	1.19
	6.0	2.86
	20	9.52
Seven servings	0.2	0.33
	2.5	4.17
	6.0	10.00
	20	33.33

[a] Shaded cells indicate where exposure exceeds the JECFA PTMI of 70 pg/kg body weight, expressed on a daily basis (2.3 pg/kg body weight per day).

In a comparison exercise, the Expert Consultation utilized the USEPA's (USEPA, 2003) suggested upper bound of the cancer risk estimation of 1×10^{-3} per picogram TEQ per kilogram body weight per day (range of cancer slope factors derived from occupational cohorts), and a hypothetical estimate of cancer deaths from dioxins was calculated as follows:

$$\text{Cancer deaths caused per million people} = [\text{Dioxins}] \times 100 \times x/7 \div 60 \times 1 \times 10^{-3} \times 10^{6}$$

where:

- [Dioxins] is the concentration of dioxins in fish (pg TEQ/g);
- 100 is the estimated fish serving size (g);
- 60 is the estimated body weight (kg); and
- x is the number of servings of fish per week.

2.5 Data on the composition of fish

Using available data, the Expert Consultation analysed the composition of fish by developing a matrix comparing levels of the LCn3PUFAs DHA and EPA with levels of total mercury and dioxins (expressed as TEQs). The matrix categorized fish species by one of four levels of each of these substances.

Four national seafood composition databases were available from France, Japan, Norway and the USA, together with one published international database. Overall, these databases provided information on the content of total fat, EPA plus DHA, total mercury and dioxins (defined to include PCDDs, PCDFs and dioxin-like PCBs). As a result of the call for data launched in the framework of this Expert Consultation in 2009, additional data were submitted by a few countries. However, these data could not be explored because they were mainly submitted as PDF files or in the form of scientific articles. The data submitted on cetacean mammals were not considered because they are outside the scope of the Expert Consultation.

Overall, the data sets included in the analyses described in this text are those from France (Leblanc *et al.*, 2006) for 45 species ($n = 750$), from Norway (National Institute of Nutrition and Seafood Research; www.nifes.no) for 17 species ($n = 3100$), from Japan (Sugiyama University, 2000; Ministry of Agriculture, Forestry and Fisheries, Japan, 2008) for 22 species ($n = 1428$) and from the USA (M. Bolger and C. Carrington, personal communication, 2010) for 51 species ($n = 3500$), as well as an international data set (Sioen *et al.*, 2007a, b) for 33 species ($n = 34\,300$). All data sets included finfish and shellfish, except for the data set from Japan, which included finfish only. Most of the compositional data are the results of analyses, whereas some are derived from compilations, such as food composition databases. The Expert Consultation had available a total of about 14 000 analytical data for EPA plus DHA, 28 000 for mercury and 15 000 for dioxins. Three of the five data sets (French, Norwegian and USA) included compositional data that were analysed on the same sample for the different compounds considered. However, the Expert Consultation noted that data on nutrient and contaminant levels in fish are lacking for many areas of the world and that a risk–benefit analysis could be conducted only for those fish species for which data are available.

Based on these five databases, a compiled data set was created, including the content of total fat, EPA plus DHA, total mercury and dioxins for 103 fish species (see Annex). This compiled data set shows the arithmetic mean content for total fat, EPA plus DHA, total mercury and dioxins in 103 species with their taxonomic names, when available, and an indication of whether they were farmed or wild caught for three species (salmon, rainbow trout and halibut). As some data were missing for some species, it was not possible to calculate a mean for every compound for each species in the list. For the combination total mercury and EPA plus DHA, data for 96 species are available (Table 3), and for the combination dioxins and EPA plus DHA, 76 species are available (Table 4). The available data did not permit evaluation of the analytical quality of the samples in terms of analytical methods, treatment of data under the limit of detection or limit of quantification, quality assurance or influence due to sampling (i.e. regional and seasonal difference) because of lacking metadata.

However, most of the data have been peer reviewed or are derived from accredited laboratories. Nevertheless, differences in the analytical methods among the different laboratories that generated the data can have an influence on the results. However, as the compiled data set is based on a very large number of samples, the mean values are considered of sufficient quality for the purposes of this report.

Correlations between the different compounds under study were investigated. No significant correlation was found between the mercury content and content of another compound.

For fish, a significant correlation was found between:

- the fat and EPA plus DHA concentrations (correlation of 0.906, $P < 0.01$);
- the dioxin and EPA plus DHA concentrations (correlation of 0.724, $P < 0.01$);
- the dioxin and fat concentrations (correlation of 0.790, $P < 0.01$).

For shellfish, a significant correlation was found between:

- the dioxin and EPA plus DHA concentrations (correlation of 0.536, $P < 0.01$).

The Expert Consultation considered that the data set was of sufficient quality for its purposes and was sufficiently comprehensive at the species level to permit a risk–benefit analysis of fish consumption following a proposed matrix combining, for each fish species, the content of total mercury and EPA plus DHA and the content of dioxins and EPA plus DHA, as reported in Tables 3 and 4. It was noted, however, that most data originated from Europe, Japan and the USA and that data from the Southern Hemisphere and developing countries are generally lacking. The Expert Consultation considered that the tables displaying the risks and benefits as a matrix, as presented in this report, could be considered as a risk–benefit communication tool for the purpose of providing advice on nutritional and safety aspects of fish consumption to consumers at the national or regional level.

Table 3. Classification of the content of EPA plus DHA by total mercury content in 96 fin fish and shellfish species

		EPA + DHA			
		$x \leq 3$ mg/g	$3 < x \leq 8$ mg/g	$8 < x \leq 15$ mg/g	$x > 15$ mg/g
Mercury	$x \leq 0.1$ µg/g	**Fish:** butterfish; catfish; cod, Atlantic; cod, Pacific; croaker, Atlantic; haddock; pike; plaice, European; pollock; saithe; sole; tilapia **Shellfish:** clams; cockle; crawfish; cuttlefish; oysters; periwinkle; scallops; scampi; sea urchin; whelk	**Fish:** flatfish; John Dory; perch, ocean and mullet; sweetfish; wolf fish **Shellfish:** mussels; squid	**Fish:** redfish; salmon, Atlantic (wild); salmon, Pacific (wild); smelt **Shellfish:** crab, spider; swimcrab	**Fish:** anchovy; herring; mackerel; rainbow trout; salmon, Atlantic (farmed); sardines; sprat **Fish liver:** cod, Atlantic (liver); saithe (liver) **Shellfish:** crab (brown meat)
	$0.1 < x \leq 0.5$ µg/g	**Fish:** anglerfish; catshark; dab; grenadier; grouper; gurnard; hake; ling; lingcod and scorpionfish; Nile perch; pout; skate/ray; snapper, porgy and sheepshead; tuna, yellowfin; tusk; whiting **Shellfish:** lobster; lobster, American	**Fish:** bass, freshwater; carp; perch, freshwater; scorpion fish; tuna; tuna, albacore **Shellfish:** crab; lobster, Norway; lobsters, spiny	**Fish:** bass, saltwater; bluefish; goatfish; halibut, Atlantic (farmed); halibut, Greenland; mackerel, horse; mackerel, Spanish; seabass; seabream; tilefish, Atlantic; tuna, skipjack	**Fish:** eel; mackerel, Pacific; sablefish
	$0.5 < x \leq 1$ µg/g	**Fish:** marlin; orange roughy; tuna, bigeye	**Fish:** mackerel, king; shark	**Fish:** alfonsino	**Fish:** tuna, Pacific bluefin
	$x > 1$ µg/g		**Fish:** swordfish		

Table 4. Classification of the content of EPA + DHA by dioxin content in 76 fin fish and shellfish species

		EPA + DHA			
		$x \leq 3$ mg/g	$3 < x \leq 8$ mg/g	$8 < x \leq 15$ mg/g	$x > 15$ mg/g
Dioxins	$x \leq 0.5$ pg TEQ/g	**Fish:** anglerfish; catshark; cod, Atlantic; grenadier; haddock; hake; ling; marlin; orange roughy; pollock; pout; saithe; skate/ray; sole; tilapia; tuna, bigeye; tuna, yellowfin; tusk; whiting **Shellfish:** cockle; clams; crawfish; cuttlefish; periwinkle; scallops; scampi; sea urchin	**Fish:** flatfish; John Dory; perch, ocean and mullet; shark; sweetfish; tuna, albacore	**Fish:** redfish; salmon, Pacific (wild); tuna, skipjack	
	$0.5 < x \leq 4$ pg TEQ/g	**Fish:** catfish; dab; gurnard; plaice, European **Shellfish:** lobster; oysters; scallops; whelk	**Fish:** scorpion fish; swordfish; tuna **Shellfish:** mussels; squid	**Fish:** alfonsino; goatfish; halibut, Atlantic (farmed); halibut, Greenland; mackerel, horse; salmon, Atlantic (wild); seabass; seabream	**Fish:** anchovy; herring; mackerel; mackerel, Pacific; rainbow trout (farmed); salmon, Atlantic (farmed); tuna, Pacific bluefin **Shellfish:** crab (brown meat)
	$4 < x \leq 8$ pg TEQ/g			**Shellfish:** crab, spider	**Fish:** sardines; sprat
	$x > 8$ pg TEQ/g			**Fish:** bluefish	**Fish:** eel **Fish liver:** cod, Atlantic (liver); saithe (liver)

2.6 Risk–benefit comparison

The Expert Consultation developed a classification system to separate fish species by the content of LCn3PUFAs (EPA plus DHA) and methylmercury or by LCn3PUFAs and dioxins with the purpose of making distinctions between types of fish and their effects on health. The choices of the cut-offs of the categories were based on typical concentrations of EPA plus DHA in different fish species and existing health-based guidance levels for methylmercury and dioxins.

In the compiled data set (Table 3), the mercury content is provided as total mercury instead of methylmercury, and the Expert Consultation assumed that for the purposes of risk–benefit comparison, 100 percent of total mercury is present as methylmercury.

Four categories were developed for methylmercury (Table 3: ≤0.1 µg/g wet weight of fish, >0.1 to ≤0.5 µg/g, >0.5 to ≤1 µg/g and >1 µg/g). The median values in each of the first three categories (0.05 µg/g, 0.3 µg/g, 0.75 µg/g) and 1.5 µg/g for >1 µg/g were used to calculate the intake dose (Sioen *et al.*, 2007a, b).

Similarly, four categories were developed for LCn3PUFAs, expressed as the sum of EPA plus DHA (Table 3): ≤3 mg/g wet weight of fish, >3 to ≤8 mg/g, >8 to ≤15 mg/g and >15 mg/g. The median values in each of the first three categories (1.5, 5.5 and 11.5 mg/g, respectively), and 20 mg/g for higher than 15 mg/g were used to calculate the intake dose.

Whereas the Expert Consultation recognized that multiple different LCn3PUFAs are present in fish, for this exercise, EPA plus DHA data were used to represent LCn3PUFAs, because it was considered that the evidence in the literature was most robust for these specific fatty acids. The Expert Consultation also decided to use an average estimate of the ratio of DHA to EPA plus DHA of 0.67 (i.e. 2:1 DHA to EPA).

For dioxins (Table 4), four categories were developed: ≤0.5 (median 0.2), >0.5 to ≤4 (median 2.5), >4 to ≤ 8 (median 6) and >8 (median 20) pg TEQ/g.

2.6.1 Neurodevelopment in newborns and infants

Table 5a–d shows the effects on child IQ as a result of the child's mother consuming one, two, four or seven servings of fish per week with different EPA plus DHA and methylmercury concentrations.

Table 5. Estimated changes in child IQ resulting from the child's mother having consumed fish with different methylmercury and EPA plus DHA contents at one, two, four and seven servings per week[a]

(a) One serving per week

			EPA + DHA			
			$x \leq 3$ mg/g	$3 < x \leq 8$ mg/g	$8 < x \leq 15$ mg/g	$x > 15$ mg/g
		Median	2	5.5	11.5	20
Methylmercury	$x \leq 0.1$ µg/g	0.05	−0.02, −0.08 +0.77	−0.02, −0.08 +2.1	−0.02, −0.08 +4.4	−0.02, −0.08 +5.8
	$0.1 < x \leq 0.5$ µg/g	0.3	−0.12, −0.47 +0.77	−0.12, −0.47 +2.1	−0.12, −0.47 +4.4	−0.12, −0.47 +5.8
	$0.5 < x \leq 1$ µg/g	0.75	−0.30, −1.2 +0.77	−0.30, −1.2 +2.1	−0.30, −1.2 +4.4	−0.30, −1.2 +5.8
	$x > 1$ µg/g	1.5	−0.60, −2.3 +0.77	−0.60, −2.3 +2.1	−0.60, −2.3 +4.4	−0.60, −2.3 +5.8

(b) Two servings per week

			EPA + DHA			
			$x \leq 3$ mg/g	$3 < x \leq 8$ mg/g	$8 < x \leq 15$ mg/g	$x > 15$ mg/g
		Median	2	5.5	11.5	20
Methylmercury	$x \leq 0.1$ µg/g	0.05	−0.04, 0.2 +1.5	−0.04, −0.2 +4.2	−0.04, −0.2 +5.8	−0.04, −0.2 +5.8
	$0.1 < x \leq 0.5$ µg/g	0.3	−0.2, −0.9 +1.5	−0.2, −0.9 +4.2	−0.2, −0.9 +5.8	−0.2, −0.9 +5.8
	$0.5 < x \leq 1$ µg/g	0.75	−0.6, −2.3 +1.5	−0.6, −2.3 +4.2	−0.6, −2.3 +5.8	−0.6, −2.3 +5.8
	$x > 1$ µg/g	1.5	−1.2, −4.7 +1.5	−1.2, −4.7 +4.2	−1.2, −4.7 +5.8	−1.2, −4.7 +5.8

(c) Four servings per week

			EPA + DHA			
			$x \leq 3$ mg/g	$3 < x \leq 8$ mg/g	$8 < x \leq 15$ mg/g	$x > 15$ mg/g
		Median	2	5.5	11.5	20
Methylmercury	$x \leq 0.1$ µg/g	0.05	−0.08, −0.31 +3.1	−0.08, −0.31 +5.8	−0.08, −0.31 +5.8	−0.08, −0.31 +5.8
	$0.1 < x \leq 0.5$ µg/g	0.3	−0.48, −1.9 +3.1	−0.48, −1.9 +5.8	−0.48, −1.9 +5.8	−0.48, −1.9 +5.8
	$0.5 < x \leq 1$ µg/g	0.75	−1.2, −4.7 +3.1	−1.2, −4.7 +5.8	−1.2, −4.7 +5.8	−1.2, −4.7 +5.8
	$x > 1$ µg/g	1.5	−2.4, −9.3 +3.1	−2.4, −9.3 +5.8	−2.4, −9.3 +5.8	−2.4, −9.3 +5.8

(d) Seven servings per week

			EPA + DHA			
			$x \leq 3$ mg/g	$3 < x \leq 8$ mg/g	$8 < x \leq 15$ mg/g	$x > 15$ mg/g
		Median	2	5.5	11.5	20
Methylmercury	$x \leq 0.1$ µg/g	0.05	−0.14, −0.5 +5.4	−0.14, −0.5 +5.8	−0.14, −0.5 +5.8	−0.14, −0.5 +5.8
	$0.1 < x \leq 0.5$ µg/g	0.3	−0.84, −3.3 +5.4	−0.84, −3.3 +5.8	−0.84, −3.3 +5.8	−0.84, −3.3 +5.8
	$0.5 < x \leq 1$ µg/g	0.75	−2.1, −8.2 +5.4	−2.1, −8.2 +5.8	−2.1, −8.2 +5.8	−2.1, −8.2 +5.8
	$x > 1$ µg/g	1.5	−4.2, −16.3 +5.4	−4.2, −16.3 +5.8	−4.2, −16.3 +5.8	−4.2, −16.3 +5.8

[a] Fish serving size was estimated to be 100 g. Ratio of DHA to EPA + DHA was assumed to be 0.67. Maternal body weight was assumed to be 60 kg. The numbers in the upper row in each cell (red) are estimates of IQ points lost from methylmercury exposure, with the lower value of the two values calculated using the central estimate of −0.18 and the higher value calculated using the upper-bound estimate of −0.7. The number in the lower row in each cell (green) is the estimate of IQ points gained from DHA exposure using the coefficient of 4 IQ points for 100 mg of DHA intake. The maximum positive effect from DHA was estimated at 5.8 points. Yellow shaded cells represent the estimates where the net effect on child IQ, using the upper-bound estimate for methylmercury, is negative.

Below are examples of how the values were calculated when one serving of fish is consumed per week. For fish with a methylmercury concentration below 0.1 µg/g, the median content of 0.05 µg/g was multiplied by the serving size of 100 g to determine the absolute methylmercury dose consumed per serving. This value was multiplied by the number of servings per week ($x = 1$) and then divided by 7 to obtain the absolute daily dose. This value was further divided by the maternal body weight of 60 kg to obtain the daily dose per kilogram of body weight, which was then converted to change in hair mercury concentration by multiplying by a factor of 9.3. The result was multiplied by a coefficient of −0.18 or −0.7 to obtain the estimated change in IQ of −0.02 or −0.08, as shown in Table 5a. This calculation can be summarized as:

$$\text{IQ points gained} = [\text{MeHg}] \times 100(x/7) \div 60 \times 9.3 \times (-0.18 \text{ or } -0.7)$$

where:

- [MeHg] is the concentration of methylmercury in fish (µg/g);
- 100 is the estimated fish serving size (g);
- x is the number of servings of fish per week (7 days);
- 60 is the estimated maternal body weight (kg);
- 9.3 is the correlation between maternal methylmercury intake and maternal hair mercury level;
- −0.18 is the central estimate of IQ points gained per microgram per gram hair mercury gained; and
- −0.7 is the upper-bound estimate of IQ points gained per microgram per gram hair mercury gained.

Similarly, for fish that has an EPA plus DHA concentration greater than 3 and less than or equal to 8 mg/g, a median of 5.5 mg/g was taken and multiplied by the serving size of 100 g to determine the absolute EPA plus DHA dose consumed per serving. This value was multiplied by the number of servings per week ($x = 1$) and then divided by 7 to obtain the absolute daily dose. This calculation was followed by multiplying by a factor of 0.67 to convert to DHA only and converted to IQ changes by multiplying by a coefficient of 0.04 using the assumption of 4 IQ points per 100 mg of DHA to obtain the estimated change in IQ of 2.1, as shown in Table 5a. This calculation can be summarized as:

$$\text{IQ points gained} = [\text{EPA} + \text{DHA}] \times 100 \times 0.67 \times (x/7) \times 0.04$$

where:

- [EPA + DHA] is the total concentration of EPA plus DHA in fish (mg/g);
- 100 is the estimated fish serving size (g);
- 0.67 is the factor used to estimate DHA concentration from [EPA + DHA];
- x is the number of servings of fish per week; and
- 0.04 is the coefficient relating IQ points gained to milligrams of DHA intake per day.

The results demonstrate that for the central estimate of −0.18 IQ point decrease per microgram per gram mercury in maternal hair, the positive IQ effects of DHA always outweigh the negative IQ effects of methylmercury, including for consumption of fish with a methylmercury content above 1 µg/g, even at the highest consumption frequency of seven servings per week.

The results also demonstrate that for the upper limit estimate of −0.70 IQ point decrease per microgram per gram mercury in maternal hair, the positive effects of DHA on IQ continue to outweigh the negative effects of methylmercury on IQ in most fish categories. For consumption of fish at one and two servings per week, the negative effect of methylmercury was higher in only three categories of fish, as marked yellow in Table 5 a) and b). For consumption of fish at seven servings per week, the negative effect of mercury was higher than the positive effects of DHA for any fish that contained more than 0.5 µg/g of methylmercury.

2.6.2 Comparison of the effects of methylmercury and DHA on children's IQ: results and discussion

Based on a quantitative risk–benefit analysis of the effects of maternal fish consumption on neurodevelopment in newborns and infants, the Expert Consultation determined the following:

1) Using central estimates for benefits of DHA and for harm from mercury, the neurodevelopmental risks of not eating fish exceed the risks of eating fish for all frequencies of consumption evaluated (range: 1–7 100 g servings per week) and all categories of fish evaluated (median ranges: 2–20 mg/g EPA + DHA and 0.05–1.5 µg/g methylmercury).

2) Using an upper bound for harm of mercury and a central estimate for benefit of DHA, the neurodevelopmental risks of not eating fish exceed the risks of eating fish for all frequencies of consumption evaluated (range: 1–7 100 g servings per week) and all categories of fish evaluated (median range: 2–20 mg/g EPA + DHA) when methylmercury levels are lower than 0.5 µg/g. When methylmercury levels are higher than this, the neurodevelopmental risks of not eating fish may no longer exceed the risks of eating fish, depending on the combination of EPA plus DHA levels, methylmercury levels and frequency of consumption. For example, when two servings per week are consumed with EPA plus DHA levels in the range from >3 to ≤8 mg/g, the neurodevelopmental risks of eating fish exceed the risks of not eating fish when methylmercury exceeds 1 µg/g. At four servings per week, the neurodevelopmental risks of eating fish exceed the risks of not eating fish when the fish contains greater than 1 µg/g methylmercury; and at seven servings per week, the neurodevelopmental risks of eating fish exceed the risks of not eating fish when fish contains greater than 0.5 µg/g methylmercury, for all the scenarios examined.

Conclusions:

1) The Expert Consultation finds the evidence convincing that maternal fish consumption contributes to optimal neurodevelopment in their offspring.

2) With a central estimate of methylmercury risk, neurodevelopmental risks of not eating fish exceed risks of eating fish for up to at least seven 100 g servings per week and methylmercury levels up to at least 1 µg/g.

3) With an upper estimate of methylmercury risk, neurodevelopmental risks of not eating fish exceed risks of eating fish for up to at least seven 100 g servings per week for all fish containing less than 0.5 µg/g methylmercury and for up to at least two servings per week for fish with greater than 8 mg/g EPA plus DHA and up to 1 µg/g methylmercury.

4) Neurodevelopmental benefits of fish consumption are reduced by methylmercury contamination, and reducing anthropogenic mercury contamination in fish would result in even greater neurodevelopmental benefits from fish consumption.

2.6.3 Mortality from coronary heart disease

Table 6a–d shows the effects on mortality as a result of consuming one, two, four or seven servings of fish per week with different EPA plus DHA and dioxin concentrations.

Table 6. Estimated changes in mortality per million people from consuming fish with different dioxin and EPA plus DHA contents at one, two, four and seven 100 g servings per week[a]

(a) One serving per week

			EPA + DHA			
			$x \leq 3$ mg/g	$3 < x \leq 8$ mg/g	$8 < x \leq 15$ mg/g	$x > 15$ mg/g
		Median	2	5.5	11.5	20
Dioxins	$x \leq 1$ pg/g	0.2	+50 −4550	+50 −12 500	+50 −26 200	+50 −39 800
	$1 < x \leq 4$ pg/g	2.5	+600 −4550	+600 −12 500	+600 −26 200	+600 −39 800
	$4 < x \leq 8$ pg/g	6	+1400 −4550	+1400 −12 500	+1400 −26 200	+1400 −39 800
	$x > 8$ pg/g	20	+4800 −4550	+4800 −12 500	+4800 −26 200	+4800 −39 800

(b) Two servings per week

			EPA + DHA			
			$x \leq 3$ mg/g	$3 < x \leq 8$ mg/g	$8 < x \leq 15$ mg/g	$x > 15$ mg/g
		Median	2	5.5	11.5	20
Dioxins	$x \leq 1.0$ pg/g	0.2	+100 −9100	+100 −25 000	+100 −39 800	+100 −39 800
	$1.0 < x \leq 4.0$ pg/g	2.5	+1200 −9100	+1200 −25 000	+1200 −39 800	+1200 −39 800
	$4.0 < x \leq 8.0$ pg/g	6.0	+2900 −9100	+2900 −25 000	+2900 −39 800	+2900 −39 800
	$x > 8.0$ pg/g	20.0	+9500 −9100	+9500 −25 000	+9500 −39 800	+9500 −39 800

(c) Four servings per week

			EPA + DHA			
			$x \leq 3$ mg/g	$3 < x \leq 8$ mg/g	$8 < x \leq 15$ mg/g	$x > 15$ mg/g
		Median	2	5.5	11.5	20
Dioxins	$x \leq 1.0$ pg/g	0.2	+190 −18 200	+190 −39 800	+190 −39 800	+190 −39 800
	$1.0 < x \leq 4.0$ pg/g	2.5	+2400 −18 200	+2400 −39 800	+2400 −39 800	+2400 −39 800
	$4.0 < x \leq 8.0$ pg/g	6.0	+5700 −18 200	+5700 −39 800	+5700 −39 800	+5700 −39 800
	$x > 8.0$ pg/g	20.0	+19 000 −18 200	+19 000 −39 800	+19 000 −39 800	+19 000 −39 800

(d) Seven servings per week

		EPA + DHA			
		$x \leq 3$ mg/g	$3 < x \leq 8$ mg/g	$8 < x \leq 15$ mg/g	$x > 15$ mg/g
	Median	2	5.5	11.5	20
Dioxins $x \leq 1.0$ pg/g	0.2	+330 −31 900	+330 −39 800	+330 −39 800	+330 −39 800
$1.0 < x \leq 4.0$ pg/g	2.5	+4200 −31 900	+4200 −39 800	+4200 −39 800	+4200 −39 800
$4.0 < x \leq 8.0$ pg/g	6.0	+10 000 −31 900	+10 000 −39 800	+10 000 −39 800	+10 000 −39 800
$x > 8.0$ pg/g	20.0	+33 300 −31 900	+33 300 −39 800	+33 300 −39 800	+33 300 −39 800

[a] Mean population body weight was assumed to be 60 kg. The numbers in the upper row in each cell (red) are estimates of lives lost from dioxin exposure, prepared using upper-bound estimates of risk. The numbers in the lower row in each cell (green) are the estimates of lives saved due to reduction in coronary heart disease risk from EPA + DHA intake. The maximum positive effect from EPA + DHA was estimated to occur at 250 mg/day. Yellow shaded cells represent the estimates where the net effect is negative; lives lost are greater than lives saved.

2.6.4 *Comparison of the effects of DHA and dioxins on coronary heart disease mortality: results and discussion*

Based on quantitative risk–benefit analysis of the effects of fish consumption on coronary heart disease mortality, the Expert Consultation determined the following:

1) Using central estimates for the effects of EPA plus DHA on coronary heart disease mortality, there are coronary heart disease benefits of eating fish (and coronary heart disease risks of not eating fish) for all frequencies of consumption evaluated (range: 1–7 100 g servings per week) and all categories of fish evaluated (median range: 2–20 mg/g EPA + DHA), other than for fish from the highest dioxin category (median 20 pg/g) and lowest EPA plus DHA level (median 2 mg/g).

2) Maximal benefit can be achieved by consumption of one serving per week of fish with an EPA plus DHA concentration greater than 15 mg/g, two servings per week of fish with an EPA plus DHA concentration greater than 8 but less than or equal to 15 mg/g, four servings per week of fish with an EPA plus DHA concentration greater than 3 but less than or equal to 8 mg/g, and seven servings per week of fish with an EPA plus DHA concentration less than or equal to 3 mg/g. However, risks are lowered by any level of fish consumption evaluated (up to seven 100 g servings per week), except for the combination of low EPA plus DHA (≤ 3 mg/g) and dioxin concentration greater than 8 pg/g.

3) In the worst case, at seven servings per week, established coronary heart disease benefits are outweighed by theoretical dioxin risks when dioxin concentrations are in the highest category (>8 pg/g). However, the Expert Consultation noted that, based on available data on dioxin levels, only a small proportion of fish have dioxin levels in this category.

Conclusions:

1) The Expert Consultation finds the evidence convincing that fish consumption lowers coronary heart disease mortality in the general population.

2) Moderate consumption of fatty fish (one or two 100 g servings per week) appears to provide maximum benefit, but risks are lowered by any level of fish consumption evaluated (up to seven 100 g servings per week) unless very high dioxin levels are present.

3) In general, when considering an upper estimate for theoretical increased cancer incidence from dioxins in fish, the defined benefits of fish consumption from reduction of coronary heart disease mortality exceeds any hypothetical cancer risk.

3. SUMMARY OF FINDINGS

3.1 Consumption of fish, LCn3PUFAs, methylmercury and dioxins in women of childbearing age, pregnant women and nursing mothers

There is *convincing* evidence that:

- LCn3PUFAs (DHA) are important for optimal brain development during gestation and infancy;
- maternal fish consumption during gestation and nursing lowers the risk of suboptimal brain development in their children; and
- maternal methylmercury exposure during gestation increases the risk of suboptimal brain development in their children.

There is *probable* evidence that:

- higher maternal body burden of total dioxins plus non-dioxin-like PCBs during gestation increases the risk of suboptimal brain development in their children.

There is *possible* evidence that:

- higher maternal body burden of dioxins during gestation increases the risk of suboptimal brain development in their children.

Based on quantitative risk–benefit analysis of DHA and methylmercury, the neurodevelopmental risks of not eating fish exceed the risks of eating fish under most circumstances evaluated:

- Optimal health benefits of fish consumption can be achieved by maximizing LCn3PUFA intake and minimizing methylmercury exposure.
- Frequency, amount and choice of fish species consumed are important in maximizing the net benefits.
- In all circumstances, neurodevelopmental benefits of fish consumption are reduced by exposure to methylmercury. In some circumstances, there may be net harm.
- Reducing anthropogenic methylmercury contamination of fish would result in even greater net neurodevelopmental benefits of fish consumption.

The evidence is currently *insufficient* to derive a dose–response relationship between dietary dioxins and neurodevelopment. This lack of a dose–response relationship limits quantitative risk–benefit analysis for the neurodevelopmental effects of DHA intake or fish consumption versus dioxin exposure. The evidence allows the following qualitative conclusions:

- Health effects of dioxins are strongly related to body burden, which accrues over months and years. The current PTMI is not applicable to evaluating the health effects of a single serving of fish.
- At levels of maternal dioxin exposure (from fish and other dietary sources) that do not exceed the PTMI, neurodevelopmental risk is negligible.
- At levels of maternal dioxin exposure (from fish and other dietary sources) that exceed the PTMI, neurodevelopmental risk may no longer be negligible.
- Reducing anthropogenic contamination of fish by dioxins would result in even greater net neurodevelopmental benefits of fish consumption.

Levels of nutrients in fish, including LCn3PUFAs, and contaminants in fish, including methylmercury and especially dioxins, can have large regional differences. Therefore, it is critical that national and regional authorities have specific information on levels of nutrients and contaminants in fish consumed in their region.

3.2 Consumption of fish, LCn3PUFAs, methylmercury and dioxins in the general adult population

There is *convincing* evidence that:

- fish consumption and EPA plus DHA intake lower the risk of coronary heart disease mortality; and
- high dioxin exposure increases the risk of cancer.

There is *insufficient to possible* evidence that:

- methylmercury exposure increases the risk of coronary heart disease.

There is *insufficient* evidence that:

- typical levels of dietary dioxins (such as seen in fish and other dietary sources) increase the risk of cancer.

Based on quantitative analysis using central estimates for EPA plus DHA benefits:

- risk of coronary heart disease mortality is significantly increased by not eating fish.

The current evidence is not sufficient to conclude that methylmercury causes coronary heart disease. This lack of evidence limits quantitative risk–benefit analysis for the effects of fish consumption or EPA plus DHA intake versus methylmercury exposure on coronary heart disease.

Based on quantitative risk–benefit analysis using central estimates for EPA plus DHA benefits and theoretical upper estimate of cancer risks from dioxins:

- coronary heart disease mortality benefits exceed theoretical upper-estimate cancer risks for all frequencies and categories of fish consumption and dioxin exposures evaluated, other than in the combination of very low EPA plus DHA and very high dioxin concentrations, a combination that was not found in the fish composition data available to the Expert Consultation.

4. RESEARCH PRIORITIES AND DATA GAPS

- Research should focus on the benefits of fish consumption and of the nutrients in fish at different life stages.
- Research should focus on strategies for establishing healthy eating patterns, including fish consumption, for later life.
- Member countries should be encouraged to generate representative data on levels of long-chain omega-3 fatty acids (LCn3PUFAs), mercury and dioxins in fish species in the form consumed in their respective countries.

5. CONCLUSIONS AND RECOMMENDATIONS

5.1 Conclusions

- Consumption of fish provides energy, protein and a range of essential nutrients.
- Eating fish is part of the cultural traditions of many peoples. In some populations, fish is a major source of food and essential nutrients.
- Among the general adult population, consumption of fish, particularly fatty fish, lowers the risk of coronary heart disease mortality. There is an absence of probable or convincing evidence of coronary heart disease risks of methylmercury. Potential cancer risks of dioxins are well below established coronary heart disease benefits.
- Among women of childbearing age, pregnant women and nursing mothers, considering benefits of DHA versus risks of methylmercury, fish consumption lowers the risk of suboptimal neurodevelopment in their offspring compared with not eating fish in most circumstances evaluated.
- At levels of maternal dioxin exposure (from fish and other dietary sources) that do not exceed the PTMI, neurodevelopmental risk is negligible. At levels of maternal dioxin exposure (from fish and other dietary sources) that exceed the PTMI, neurodevelopmental risk may no longer be negligible.
- Among infants, young children and adolescents, evidence is insufficient to derive a quantitative framework of health risks and benefits. However, healthy dietary patterns that include fish consumption and are established early in life influence dietary habits and health during adult life.

5.2 Recommendations

To minimize risks in target populations, the Expert Consultation recommends that Member States should:

- acknowledge fish as an important food source of energy, protein and a range of essential nutrients and fish consumption as part of the cultural traditions of many peoples;
- emphasize the benefits of fish consumption on reducing coronary heart disease mortality (and the risks of mortality from coronary heart disease associated with not eating fish) for the general adult population;
- emphasize the net neurodevelopmental benefits to offspring of fish consumption by women of childbearing age, particularly pregnant women and nursing mothers, and the neurodevelopmental risks of not consuming fish to offspring of such women;
- develop, maintain and improve existing databases on specific nutrients and contaminants, particularly methylmercury and dioxins, in fish consumed in their region;
- develop and evaluate risk management and communication strategies that both minimize risks and maximize benefits from eating fish.

6. REFERENCES

Ahlquist, M., Bengtsson, C., Lapidus, L., Bergdahl, I.A. & Schutz, A. 1999. Serum mercury concentration in relation to survival, symptoms, and diseases: results from the prospective population study of women in Gothenburg, Sweden. *Acta Odontologica Scandinavica*, 57:168–174.

Albert, C.M., Hennekens, C.H., O'Donnell, C.J., Ajani, U.A., Carey, V.J., Willett, W.C., Ruskin, J.N. & Manson, J.E. 1998. Fish consumption and risk of sudden cardiac death. *JAMA: Journal of the American Medical Association*, 279:23–28.

Albert, C.M., Campos, H., Stampfer, M.J., Ridker, P.M., Manson, J.E., Willett, W.C. & Ma, J. 2002. Blood levels of long-chain n-3 fatty acids and the risk of sudden death. *New England Journal of Medicine*, 346:1113–1118.

Arnold, S. M., Lynn, T. V., Verbrugge, L.A. & Middaugh, J.P. 2005. Human biomonitoring to optimize fish consumption advice: reducing uncertainty when evaluating benefits and risks. *American Journal of Public Health*, 95(3):393–397.

Axelrad, D.A., Bellinger, D.C., Ryan, L.M. & Woodruff, T.J. 2007. Dose–response relationship of prenatal mercury exposure and IQ: an integrative analysis of epidemiologic data. *Environmental Health Perspectives*, 115(4):609–615.

Bakalar, N. 2007. Nutrition: Study questions limits on fish in pregnancy. *The New York Times*, 27 February. Available at: www.nytimes.com/2007/02/27/health/27nutr.html?scp=1&sq=bakalar%2027%20february%202007%20fish%20pregnancy&st=cse

Bhavsar, S.P., Hayton, A., Reiner, E.J. & Jackson, D.A. 2007. Estimating dioxin-like polychlorinated biphenyl toxic equivalents from total polychlorinated biphenyl measurements in fish. *Environmental Science & Technology*, 41(9):3096–3102. Buozan C *et al.* 2005. A quantitative analysis of fish consumption and stroke risk. *American Journal of Preventive Medicine*, 29(4):347–352.

Bouzan, C., Cohen, J.T., Connor, W.E., Kris-Etherton, P.M., Gray, G.M. Konig, A., Lawrence, R.S., Savitz, D.A. & Teutsch S.M. 2005. A quantitative analysis of fish consumption and stroke risk. *American Journal of Preventive Medicine*, 29(4):347–352.

BRAFO 2010. BRAFO Methodology application to the case studies. Retrieved July 06, 2011 from: www.brafo.org/downloadattachment/6200/3216/BRAFO-16no10-Hoekstra.pdf

Budtz-Jørgensen, E., Debes, F., Weihe, P. & Grandjean, P. 2005. Adverse Mercury Effects in 7 Year Old Children Expressed as Loss in "IQ." *Report to the U.S. Environmental Protection Agency.* EPA-HQ-OAR-2002-0056-6046. Available: www.regulations.gov (Accessed 29 June 2011)

Budtz-Jørgensen, E.P., Grandjean, P. & Weihe, P. 2007. Separation of risks and benefits of seafood intake. *Environmental Health Perspectives*, 115(3):323–327.

Burr, M.L., Fehily, A.M., Gilbert, J.F., Rogers, S., Holliday, R.M., Sweetnam, P.M., Elwood, P.C. & Deadman, N.M. 1989. Effects of changes in fat, fish, and fibre intakes on death and myocardial reinfarction: diet and reinfarction trial (DART). *Lancet*, 2(8666):757–761.

Burr, M.L., Ashfield-Watt, P.A., Dunstan, F.D., Fehily, A.M., Breay, P., Ashton, T., Zotos, P.C., Haboubi, N.A. & Elwood, P.C. 2003. Lack of benefit of dietary advice to men with angina: results of a controlled trial. *European Journal of Clinical Nutrition*, 57:193–200.

Carrington, C.D. & Bolger, P.M. 2000. A pooled analysis of the Iraqi and Seychelles methylmercury studies. *Human and Ecological Risk Assessment*, 6:323–340.

Clarkson, T.W. & Magos, L. 2006. The toxicology of mercury and its chemical compounds. *Critical Reviews in Toxicology*, 36:609–662.

Cohen, J.T., Bellinger, D.C., Connor, W.E., Kris-Etherton, P.M., Lawrence, R.S., Savitz, D.A., Shaywitz, B.A., Teutsch, S.M. & Gray, G.M. 2005a. A quantitative risk–benefit analysis of changes in population fish consumption. *American Journal of Preventive Medicine*, 29(4):325–334.

Cohen, J.T., Bellinger, D.C. & Shaywitz, B.A. 2005b. A quantitative analysis of prenatal methyl mercury exposure and cognitive development. *American Journal of Preventive Medicine*, 29(4):353–366.

Cohen, J.T., Bellinger D.C., Connor, W.E. & Shaywitz, B.A. 2005c. A quantitative analysis of prenatal intake of n-3 polyunsaturated fatty acids and cognitive development. *American Journal of Preventive Medicine*, 29(4):366–374.

Colombo, J., Kannass, K.N., Shaddy, D.J., Kundurthi, S., Maikranz, J.M., Anderson, C.J., Blaga, O.M. & Carlson, S.E. 2004. Maternal DHA and the development of attention in infancy and toddlerhood. *Child Development*, 75:1254–1267.

Crump, K.S., Kjellstrom, T., Shipp, A.M., Silvers, A. & Stewart, A. 1998. Influence of prenatal mercury exposure upon scholastic and psychological test performance: benchmark analysis of a New Zealand cohort. *Risk Analysis*, 18:701–713.

Daniels, J.L., Longnecker, M.P., Rowland, A.S. & Golding, J. 2004. Fish intake during pregnancy and early cognitive development of offspring. *Epidemiology*, 15:394–402.

Davidson, P.W., Myers, G.J., Cox, C., Axtell, C., Shamlaye, C., Sloane-Reeves, J., Cernichiari, E., Needham, L., Choi, A., Wang, Y., Berlin, M. & Clarkson, T.W. 1998. Effects of prenatal and postnatal methylmercury exposure from fish consumption on neurodevelopment: outcomes at 66 months of age in the Seychelles child development study. *JAMA: Journal of the American Medical Association*, 280:701–707.

Davidson, P.W., Palumbo, D., Myers, G.J., Cox, C., Shamlaye, C.F., Sloane-Reeves, J., Cernichiari, E., Wilding, G.E. & Clarkson, T.W. 2000. Neurodevelopmental outcomes of Seychellois children from the pilot cohort at 108 months following prenatal exposure to methylmercury from a maternal fish diet. *Environmental Research*, 84(1):1–11.

Davidson, P.W., Myers, G.J., Cox, C., Wilding, G.E., Shamlaye, C.F., Huang, L.S., Cernichiari, E., Sloane-Reeves, J. Palumbo, D. & Clarkson, T.W. 2006. Methylmercury and neurodevelopment: longitudinal analysis of the Seychelles child development cohort. *Neurotoxicology and Teratology*, 28(5):529–535.

Davidson, P.W., Strain, J.J., Myers, G.J., Thurston, S.W., Bonham, M.P., Shamlaye, C.F., Stokes-Riner, A., Wallace, J.M., Robson, P.J., Duffy, E.M., Georger, L.A., Sloane-Reeves, J., Cernichiari, E., Canfield, R.L., Cox, C., Huang, L.S., Janciuras, J. & Clarkson, T.W. 2008. Neurodevelopmental effects of maternal nutritional status and exposure to methylmercury from eating fish during pregnancy. *Neurotoxicology*, 29(5):767–775.

Daviglus, M.L., Stamler, J., Orencia, A.J., Dyer, A.R., Liu, K., Greenland, P., Walsh, M.K., Morris, D. & Shekelle, R.B. 1997. Fish consumption and the 30-year risk of fatal myocardial infarction. *New England Journal of Medicine*, 336:1046–1053.

Debes, F.E., Budtz-Jørgensen, P., Weihe, P., White, R.F. & Grandjean, P. 2006. Impact of prenatal methylmercury exposure on neurobehavioural function at age 14 years. *Neurotoxicology and Teratology*, 28:363–375.

Dickhoff, W., Collier, T. & Varanasi, U. 2007. The seafood dilemma—a way forward. *Fisheries*, 32(5):244–246.

Dolecek, T.A. & Granditis, G. 1991. Dietary polyunsaturated fatty acids and mortality in the Multiple Risk Factor Intervention Trial (MRFIT). *World Review of Nutrition*, 66:205–216.

EFSA Scientific Committee 2010. Scientific opinion: Guidance on human health risk–benefit assessment of foods. *EFSA Journal*, 8(7):1673 (www.efsa.europa.eu/de/scdocs/doc/1673.pdf).

Egeland, G.M. & Middaugh, J.P. 1997. Balancing fish consumption benefits with mercury exposure. *Science*, 278(5345):1904–1905.

FAO 2010. *Fats and fatty acids in human nutrition. Report of an expert consultation.* Rome, Food and Agriculture Organization of the United Nations (FAO Food and Nutrition Paper 91; www.fao.org/docrep/013/i1953e/i1953e00.pdf).

FAO/WHO 2002. *Evaluation of certain food additives and contaminants: fifty-seventh report of the Joint FAO/WHO Expert Committee on Food Additives.* Geneva, World Health Organization (WHO Technical Report Series, No. 909).

FAO/WHO 2004. *Evaluation of certain food additives and contaminants: sixty-first report of the Joint FAO/WHO Expert Committee on Food Additives.* Geneva, World Health Organization (WHO Technical Report Series, No. 922).

FAO/WHO 2007. *Evaluation of certain food additives and contaminants: sixty-seventh report of the Joint FAO/WHO Expert Committee on Food Additives.* Geneva, World Health Organization (WHO Technical Report Series, No. 940).

FAO/WHO 2010. *Codex Alimentarius Commission procedural manual*, 19th ed. Rome, World Health Organization and Food and Agriculture Organization of the United Nations, Joint FAO/WHO Food Standards Programme (www.codexalimentarius.net/web/procedural_manual.jsp).

Folsom, A.R. & Demissie, Z. 2004. Fish intake, marine omega-3 fatty acids, and mortality in a cohort of postmenopausal women. *American Journal of Epidemiology*, 160:1005–1010.

Foran, J.A., Good, D.H., Carpenter, D.O., Hamilton, M.C., Knuth, B.A. & Schwager, S.J. 2005. Quantitative analysis of the benefits and risks of consuming farmed and wild salmon. *Journal of Nutrition*, 135(11):2639–2643.

Foran, J.A., Carpenter, D.O., Good, D.H., Hamilton, M.C., Hites, R.A., Knuth, B.A. & Schwager, S.J. 2006. Risks and benefits of seafood consumption. *American Journal of Preventive Medicine*, 30(5):438–439.

Fraser, G.E., Sabate, J., Beeson, W.L. & Strahan, T.M. 1992. A possible protective effect of nut consumption on risk of coronary heart disease. The Adventist Health Study. *Archives of Internal Medicine*, 152:1416–1424.

Ginsberg, G. & Toal, B.F. 2009. Quantitative approach for incorporating methylmercury risks and omega-3 fatty acid benefits in developing species-specific fish consumption advice. *Environmental Health Perspectives*, 117(2):267–275.

Gladyshev, M.I., Sushchik, N.N., Anishchenco, A.V., Makhutova, O.N., Kalachova, G.S. & Gribovskya, I.V. 2009. Benefit–risk ratio of food fish intake as the source of essential fatty acids vs. heavy metals: a case study of Siberian grayling from the Yenisei River. *Food Chemistry*, 115(2):545–550.

Gochfeld, M. & Burger, J. 2005. Good fish/bad fish: a composite benefit–risk by dose curve. *Neurotoxicology*, 26(4):511–520.

Grandjean, P., Weihe, P. & White, R.F. 1995. Milestone development in infants exposed to methylmercury from human milk. *Neurotoxicology*, 16:27–33.

Grandjean, P., Weihe, P., White, R.F., Debes, F., Araki, S., Yokoyama, K., Murata, K., Sorensen, N., Dahl, R. & Jorgensen, P.J. 1997. Cognitive deficit in 7-year-old children with prenatal exposure to methylmercury. *Neurotoxicology and Teratology*, 19:417–428.

GISSI-Prevenzione Investigators (Gruppo Italiano per lo Studio della Sopravvivenza nell'Infarto miocardico). 1999. Dietary supplementation with n-3 polyunsaturated fatty acids and vitamin E after myocardial infarction: results of the GISSI-Prevenzione trial. *Lancet*, 354(9177):47–55.

Guallar, E., Sanz-Gallardo, M.I., van't Veer, P., Bode, A., Gomez-Aracena, J. & Kark, J.D. 2002. Mercury, fish oils, and the risk of myocardial infarction. *New England Journal of Medicine*, 347:1747N–1754N.

Guevel, M.R., Sirot, V., Volatier, J.L. and LeBlanc, J.C. 2008. A risk–benefit analysis of French high fish consumption: a QALY approach. *Risk Analysis*, 28(1):37–48.

Haggqvist, B., Havarinasab, S., Bjorn, E. & Hultman, P. 2005. The immunosuppressive effect of methylmercury does not preclude development of autoimmunity in genetically susceptible mice. *Toxicology*, 208:149–164.

Hallgren, C.G., Hallmans, G., Jansson, J.H., Marklund, S.L., Huhtasaari, F. & Schutz, A. 2001. Markers of high fish intake are associated with decreased risk of a first myocardial infarction. *British Journal of Nutrition*, 86:397–404.

Hansen, J.C. & Gilman, A.P. 2005. Exposure of Arctic populations to methylmercury from consumption of marine food: an updated risk–benefit assessment. *International Journal of Circumpolar Health*, 64:121–136.

Harris, W.S., Mozaffarian, D., Lefevre,, M. Toner,, C.D., Colombo, J., Cunnane, S.C., Holden, J.M., Klurfeld, D.M., Morris, M.C. & Whelan, J. 2009. Towards establishing dietary reference intakes for eicosapentaenoic and docosahexaenoic acids. *Journal of Nutrition*, 139:804S–819S.

Hastings M. 2006. Disparate claims make seafood confusing. *Winston-Salem Journal*, 25 October.

Hayabuchi, H., Yoshimura, T. & Kuratsune, M. 1979. Consumption of toxic rice oil by 'yusho' patients and its relation to the clinical response and latent period. *Food Cosmet Toxicol*, 17(5):455–461.

He, K., Song, Y., Daviglus, M.L., Liu, K., Van Horn, L. Dyer, A.R. & Greenland, P. 2004a. Accumulated evidence on fish consumption and coronary heart disease mortality: a meta-analysis of cohort studies. *Circulation*, 109(22):2705–2711.

He, K., Song, Y., Daviglus, M.L., Liu, K., Van Horn, L, Dyer, A.R. Goldbourt, U. & Greenland, P. 2004b. Fish consumption and incidence of stroke: a meta-analysis of cohort studies. *Stroke*, 35:1538–1542.

Hibbeln, J.R., Davis, J.M., Steer, C.P., Emmett, I., Rogers, C., Williams, C. & Golding, J. 2007. Maternal seafood consumption in pregnancy and neurodevelopmental outcomes in childhood (ALSPAC study): an observational cohort study. *Lancet*, 369:578–585.

Hoekstra, J., Verkaik-Kloosterman, J., Rompelberg, C., van Kranen, H., Zeilmaker, M., Verhagen, H. & de Jong, N. 2008. Integrated risk–benefit analyses: method development with folic acid as example. *Food and Chemical Toxicology*, 46(3):893–909.

Hoekstra, J., Hart, A., Boobis, A., Claupein, E., Cockburn, A., Hunt, A., Knudsen, I., Richardson, D., Schilter B., Schütte, K., Torgerson, P.R. Verhagen, H., Watzl, B. & Chiodini, A. 2010. BRAFO tiered approach for benefit–risk assessment of foods. *Food and Chemical Toxicology* (in press).

Hooper, L.R.L., Thompson, R.A., Harrison, C.D., Summerbell, C.D., Ness,, A.R., Moore, H.J., Worthington, H.V., Durrington, J.P., Higgins, J.P.T., Capps, N.E., Riemersma, R.A., Ebrahim, S.B.J. & Smith, G.D. 2006. Risks and benefits of omega 3 fats for mortality, cardiovascular disease, and cancer: systematic review. *BMJ (Clinical research ed.)*, 332(7544):752–760.

Hu, F.B., Bronner, L. & Willett, W.C. 2002. Fish and omega-3 fatty acid intake and risk of coronary heart disease in women. *JAMA: Journal of the American Medical Association*, 287:1815–1821.

Huisman, M., Koopman-Esseboom, C., Fidler, V., Hadders-Algra, M., van der Paauw, C.G., Tuinstra, L.G., Weisglas-Kuperus, N., Sauer, P.J., Touwen, B.C. & Boersma, E.R. 1995. Perinatal exposure to polychlorinated biphenyls and dioxins and its effect on neonatal neurological development. *Early Human Development*, 41(2):111–127.

IARC 1997. *Polychlorinated dibenzo-para-dioxins and polychlorinated dibenzofurans*. Lyon, International Agency for Research on Cancer (IARC Monographs on the Evaluation of Carcinogenic Risks to Humans, Vol. 69).

IPCS 1990. *Methyl mercury*. Geneva, World Health Organization, International Programme on Chemical Safety (Environmental Health Criteria 101).

Itai, Y., Fujino, T., Ueno, K. & Motomatsu, Y. 2004. An epidemiological study of the incidence of abnormal pregnancy in areas heavily contaminated with methylmercury. *Environmental Science*, 11:83–97.

Jacobson, J.L. & Jacobson, S.W. 2003. Prenatal exposure to polychlorinated biphenyls and attention at school age. *Journal of Pediatrics*, 143(6):780–788.

Kjellstrom,T., Kennedy, P., Wallis, S. & Mantell, C. 1986. *Physical and mental development of children with prenatal exposure to mercury from fish. Stage 1. Preliminary tests at age 4*. Solna, National Swedish Environmental Protection Board (Report 3080).

Kjellstrom, T., Kennedy, P., Wallis, S., Stewart, A., Friberg, L., Lind, B., Witherspoon, P. & Mantell, C. 1989. *Physical and mental development of children with prenatal exposure to mercury from fish. Stage 2. Interviews and psychological tests at age 6*. Solna, National Swedish Environmental Protection Board (Report 3642).

Knuth, B. A., Connelly, N.A., Sheeshka, J. & Patterson, J. 2003. Weighing health benefit and health risk information when consuming sport-caught fish. *Risk Analysis*, 23(6):1185–1197.

Kogevinas, M. 2000 Studies of cancer in humans. *Food Additives and Contaminants*, 17 (4): 317-324.

Konig, A., Bouzan, C., Cohen, J.T., Connor, W.E., Kris-Etherton, P.M., Gray, G.M., Lawrence, R.S., Savitz, D.A. & Teutsch, S.M. 2005. A quantitative analysis of fish consumption and coronary heart disease mortality. *American Journal of Preventive Medicine*, 29(4):335–346.

Kromhout, D., Bosschieter, E.B. & de Lezenne Coulander, E.B. 1985. The inverse relation between fish consumption and 20-year mortality from coronary heart disease. *New England Journal of Medicine*, 312:1205–1209.

Kromhout, D., Feskens, E.J. & Bowles, C.H. 1995. The protective effect of a small amount of fish on coronary heart disease mortality in an elderly population. *International Journal of Epidemiology*, 24:340–345.

Kuhnlein, H.V. 1995. Benefits and risks of traditional food for Indigenous Peoples: focus on dietary intakes of Arctic men. *Canadian Journal of Physiology and Pharmacology*, 73(6):765–771.

Kuhnlein, H.V. 2003. Promoting the nutritional and cultural benefits of traditional food systems of Indigenous People. *Forum of Nutrition*, 56:222–223.

Leblanc, J.C., Volatier, J.L., Sirot, V. & Bemrah-Aouachria, N. 2006. CALIPSO. Fish and seafood consumption study and biomarker of exposure to trace elements, pollutants and omega 3. Maisons-Alfort, French Food Safety Agency (www.afssa.fr/Documents/PASER-Ra-CalipsoEN.pdf).

Leijs, M.M., Ten Tuscher, G.W., Kees, O., Van Aalderen, W.M.C., Vulsma, T., Westra, M.., Oosting, J & Koppe, J. 2008. Perinatal dioxin exposure in the Netherlands—a long-term follow-up. *International Journal of Environmental Health*, 2(3–4):429–438.

Lemaitre, R.N., King, I.B., Mozaffarian, D., Kuller, L.H. ,Tracy, R.P. & Siscovick, D.S. 2003. n-3 polyunsaturated fatty acids, fatal ischemic heart disease, and nonfatal myocardial infarction in older adults: the Cardiovascular Health Study. *American Journal of Clinical Nutrition*, 77:319–325.

Lewin, G.A., Schachter, H.M., Yuen, D., Merchant, P., Mamaladze, V. & Tsertsvadze, A. 2005. *Effects of omega-3 fatty acids on child and maternal health.* Rockville, MD, Agency for Healthcare Research and Quality (Evidence Reports/Technology Assessments, No. 118).

Lim, S., Chung, H.U., & Paek, D. 2010. Low dose mercury and heart rate variability among community residents nearby to an industrial complex in Korea. *Neurotoxicology*, 1:10–16.

Lynch , M.L., Huang, L. S., Cox, C., Strain, J.J., Myers, G. J., Bonham, M. P., Shamlaye, C. F. ,Stokes-Riner, A., Wallace, J.M.W., Duffy, E.M., Clarkson, T.W. & Davidson, P.W. 2011. Varying coefficient function models to explore interactions between maternal nutritional status and prenatal methylmercury toxicity in the Seychelles Child Development Nutrition Study. *Environmental Research*, 111(1):75–80.

Mann, J.I., Appleby, P.N., Key, T.J. & Thorogood, M. 1997. Dietary determinants of ischaemic heart disease in health conscious individuals. *Heart*, 78:450–455.

Marchioli, R., Marfisi, R.M., Borrelli, G., Chieffo, C., Franzosi, M.G., Levantesi, G., Maggioni, A.P., Nicolosi, G.L., Scarano, M., Silletta, M.G., Schweiger, C., Tavazzi, L. & Tognoni, G. 2007. Efficacy of n-3 polyunsaturated fatty acids according to clinical characteristics of patients with recent myocardial infarction: insights from the GISSI-Prevenzione Trial. *Journal of Cardiovascular Medicine* (Hagerstown, Md.), 8(Suppl. 1):S34–S37.

Martinez, M. 1992. Tissue levels of polyunsaturated fatty acids during early human development. *Journal of Pediatrics*, 120(4 Pt 2):S129–S138.

Ministry of Agriculture, Forestry and Fisheries, Japan 2008. *Surveillance on mercury and methylmercury in fish and fishery products, 2007–2008*. Tokyo, Ministry of Agriculture, Forestry and Fisheries.

Morrissey, M.T. 2006. The good, the bad, and the ugly: weighing the risks and benefits of seafood consumption. *Nutrition and Health*, 18(2):193–197.

Mozaffarian, D. & Rimm, E.B. 2006. Fish intake, contaminants, and human health—Evaluating the risks and the benefits. *JAMA: Journal of the American Medical Association*, 296(15):1885–1899.

Mozaffarian, D., Lemaitre, R.N. Kuller, L.H. Burke, G.L. Tracy, R.P. & Siscovick,D.S. 2003. Cardiac benefits of fish consumption may depend on the type of fish meal consumed: the Cardiovascular Health Study. *Circulation*, 107:1372–1377.

Mozaffarian, D., Ascherio, A., Hu, F.B., Stampfer, M.J., Willett, W.C., Siscovick, D.S. &. Rimm, E.B. 2005. Interplay between different polyunsaturated fatty acids and risk of coronary heart disease in men. *Circulation*, 111:157–164.

Murata, K., Weihe, P., Budtz-Jørgensen, E., Jørgensen, P.J. & Grandjean, P. 2004. Delayed brainstem auditory evoked potential latencies in 14-year-old children exposed to methylmercury. *Journal of Pediatrics*, 144:177–183.

Myers, G.J., Davidson, P.W., Cox, C., Shamlaye, C.F., Tanner, M.A., Choisy, O., Sloane-Reeves, J., Marsh, D., Cernichiari, E. & Choi, A. 1995a. Neurodevelopment outcomes of Seychellois children sixty-six months after in utero exposure to methylmercury from maternal fish diet: pilot study. *Neurotoxicology*, 16:639–652.

Myers, G.J., Davidson, P.W., Cox, C., Shamlaye, C.F., Tanner, M.A., Marsh, D.O., Cernichiari E., Lapham, L.W., Berlin, M. & Clarkson, T.W. 1995b. Summary of the Seychelles Child Development Study on the relationship of fetal methylmercury exposure to neurodevelopment. *Neurotoxicology*, 16:711–716.

Myers, G.J., Marsh, D.O., Cox, C., Davidson, P.W., Shamlaye, C.F., Tanner, M.A., Choi, A.,Cernichiari, E., Choisy, O. & Clarkson, T.W. 1995c. A pilot neurodevelopmental study of Seychellois children following in utero exposure to methylmercury from maternal fish diet. *Neurotoxicology*, 16:629–638.

Myers, G.J., Davidson, P.W., Cox, C., Shamlaye, C.F., Palumbo, D., Cernichiari, E., Sloane-Reeves, J., Wilding, G.E., Kost, J., Huang, L.S. & Clarkson, T.W. 2003. Prenatal methylmercury exposure from ocean fish consumption in the Seychelles Child Development Study. *Lancet*, 361:1686–1692.

Nakamura, Y., Ueshima, H., Okamura, T., Kadowaki, T., Hayakawa,, T. Kita, Y., Tamaki, S. & Okayama, A. 2005. Association between fish consumption and all-cause and cause-specific mortality in Japan: NIPPON DATA80, 1980–99. *American Journal of Medicine*, 118:239–245.

National Healthy Mothers, Healthy Babies Coalition 2007. *Experts in obstetrics and nutrition unveil seafood consumption recommendations during pregnancy.* Press release, 4 October 2007. Alexandria, VA, National Health Mothers, Healthy Babies Coalition.

Nesheim, M.C. & Yaktine, A.L. eds 2007. *Seafood choices: balancing benefits and risks*. Prepared by the Committee on Nutrient Relationships in Seafood: Selections to Balance Benefits and Risks, Food and Nutrition Board, Institute of Medicine, National Academies. Washington, DC, The National Academies Press.

Nichols, B.R., Henz K.L., Aylward, L., Hayes, S.M. & Lamb, J.C. 2007. Age-specific reference ranges for polychlorinated biphenyls (PCB) based on the NHANES 2001–2002 survey. *Journal of Toxicology and Environmental Health, Part A*, 70:1873–1877.

Oken, E., Wright, R.O., Kleinman, K.P., Bellinger, D., Amarasiriwardena, C.J. & Hu, H. 2005. Maternal fish consumption, hair mercury and infant cognition in a U.S. cohort. *Environmental Health Perspectives*, 113:1376–1380.

Oken, E., Radesky, J.S. ,Wright, R.O., Bellinger, D.C., Amarasiriwardena, C.J., & Kleinman, K.P. 2008a. Maternal fish intake during pregnancy, blood mercury levels, and child cognition at age 3 years in a US cohort. *American Journal of Epidemiology*, 167:1171–1181.

Oken, E., Østerdal, M.L., Gillman, M.W., Knudsen V.K., Halldorsson, T.I., Strøm, M. & Bellinger, D.C. 2008b. Associations of maternal fish intake during pregnancy and breastfeeding duration with attainment of developmental milestones in early childhood: a study from the Danish National Birth Cohort. *American Journal of Clinical Nutrition*, 288:789–796.

Oomen, C.M., Feskens, E.J., Rasanen, L., Fidanza, F., Nissinen, A.M., Menotti, A.M. ,Kok, F.J. & Kromhouit, D. 2000. Fish consumption and coronary heart disease mortality in Finland, Italy, and the Netherlands. *American Journal of Epidemiology*, 151:999–1006.

Osler, M., Andreasen, A.H. & Hoidrup, S. 2003. No inverse association between fish consumption and risk of death from all-causes, and incidence of coronary heart disease in middle-aged, Danish adults. *Journal of Clinical Epidemiology*, 56:274–279.

Pesatori, A.C., Consonni, D., Tironi, A., Zocchetti C, Fini, A. & Bertazzi, P.A. 1993. Cancer in a young population in a dioxin-contaminated area. *International Journal of Epidemiology* 22(6):1010-1013

Ponce, R.A., Bartell, S.M., Wong, E.Y., LaFlamme, D., Carrington, C., Lee, R.C., Patrick, D.L., Faustman, E.M. & Bolger, M. 2000. Use of quality-adjusted life year weights with dose–response models for public health decisions: a case study of the risks and benefits of fish consumption. *Risk Analysis*, 20(4):529–542.

Ponce, R.A., Wong, E.Y. & Faustman, E.M. 2001. Quality adjusted life years (QALYs) and dose–response models in environmental health policy analysis—methodological considerations. *Science of the Total Environment*, 274(1–3):79–91.

Raaschou-Nielsen, O., Pavuk, M., Leblanc, A., Dumas, P., Philippe Weber J., Olsen, A., Tjonneland, A., Overvad, K. & Olsen, J.H. 2005. Adipose organochlorine concentrations and risk of breast cancer among postmenopausal Danish women. *Cancer Epidemiology, Biomarkers and Prevention*, 14(1):67–74.

Rissanen, T., Voutilainen, S., Nyyssonen, K., Lakka, T.A. & Salonen, J.T. 2000. Fish oil–derived fatty acids, docosahexaenoic acid and docosapentaenoic acid, and the risk of acute coronary events. The Kuopio Ischaemic Heart Disease Risk Factor Study. *Circulation*, 102:2677–2679.

Ryan, L.M. 2005. Effects of Prenatal Methylmercury on Childhood IQ: A Synthesis of Three Studies. Report to the U.S. Environmental Protection Agency. EPA-HQ-OAR-2002-0056-6048 and EPA-HQ-OAR-2002-0056-6049. Available: www.regulations.gov

Sakamoto, M., Nakano, A. & Akagi, H. 2001. Declining Minamata male birth ratio associated with increased male fetal death due to heavy methylmercury pollution. *Environmental Research*, 87:92–98.

Sakamoto, M., Kubota, M., Liu, X.J., Murata, K., Nakai, K. & Satoh, H. 2004. Maternal and fetal mercury and n-3 polyunsaturated fatty acids as a risk and benefit of fish consumption to fetus. *Environmental Science & Technology*, 38(14):3860–3863.

Salonen, J.T., Seppanen, K., Lakka, T.A., Salonen, R. & Kaplan, G.A. 1995. Intake of mercury from fish, lipid peroxidation, and the risk of myocardial infarction and coronary, cardiovascular, and any death in eastern Finnish men. *Circulation*, 91:645–655.

Salonen, J.T., Seppanen, K., Nyyssonen, K., Korpela, H., Kauhanen, J. & Kantola, M. 2000. Mercury accumulation and accelerated progression of carotid atherosclerosis: a population-based prospective 4-year follow-up study in men in eastern Finland. *Atherosclerosis*, 148:265–273.

Schantz, S.L., Widholm, J.J. & Rice, D.C. 2003 Effects of PCB exposure on neuropsychological function in children. *Environmental Health Perspectives*. Mar;111(3):357-576.

Scherer, A.C., Tsuchiya, A., Younglove, L.R., Burbacher, T.M. & Faustman, E.M. 2008. Comparative analysis of state fish consumption advisories targeting sensitive populations. *Environmental Health Perspectives*, 116(12):1598–1606.

Scott, L. 2007. Group gives fishy advice to pregnant women. *Jewish World Review*, 25 October (jewishworldreview.com/1007/fishy_advice.php3).

Sidhu, K.S. 2003. Health benefits and potential risks related to consumption of fish or fish oil. *Regulatory Toxicology and Pharmacology*, 38(3):336–344.

Silbergeld, E.K., Silva, I.A. & Nyland, J.F. 2005. Mercury and autoimmunity: implications for occupational and environmental health. *Toxicology and Applied Pharmacology*, 207:282–292.

Sioen, I., De Henauw, S., Verdonck, F., Van Thuyne, N. & Van Camp, J. 2007a. Development of a nutrient database and distributions for use in a probabilistic risk–benefit analysis of human fish consumption. *Journal of Food Composition and Analysis*, 20(8):662–670.

Sioen, I., Van Camp, J., Verdonck, F., Van Thuyne, N., Willems, J. & De Henauw S. 2007b. How to use secondary data on seafood contamination for probabilistic exposure assessment purposes? Main problems and potential solutions. *Human and Ecological Risk Assessment*, 13:632–657.

Squires, S. 2006a. Good fish, bad fish; sorting seafood's benefits from risks can leave consumers floundering. *Washington Post*, 8 August, F:1.

Squires, S. 2006b. New studies give fish a clean bill of health, though questions remain. *Washington Post*, 24 October, F:8.

Squires, S. 2007. Pregnant women advised to eat fish. *Washington Post*, 4 October, A:10.

Stewart, P.W., Lonky E., Reihman, J., Pagano, J., Gump, B.B. & Darvil, T. 2008. The relationship between prenatal PCB exposure and intelligence (IQ) in 9-year-old children. *Environmental Health Perspectives*, 116(10):1416–1422.

Strain, J.J., Davidson, P.W., Bonham, M.P., Duffy, E.M., Stokes-Riner, A., Thurston, S.W., Wallace, J.M.W., Robson, P.J., Shamlaye, C.F., Georger, L.A., Sloane-Reeves, J., Cernichiari, E., Canfield, R.L., Cox, C., Huang, L.S., Janciuras, J., Myers, G. J. & Clarkson, T.W. 2008. Associations of maternal long-chain polyunsaturated fatty acids, methyl mercury, and infant development in the Seychelles Child Development Nutrition Study. *Neurotoxicology*, 29(5):776–782.

Sugiyama University 2004. *Food composition database.* (database.food.sugiyama-u.ac.jp/index_asia.php).

Tsuchiya, A., Hardy, J., Burbacher, T.M., Faustman E.M., & Marien, K. 2008. Fish intake guidelines: incorporating n-3 fatty acid intake and contaminant exposure in the Korean and Japanese communities. *American Journal of Clinical Nutrition*, 87(6):1867–1875.

Tuomisto, J.T., Tuomisto, J., Tainio,, M. Niittynen,, M., Verkasalo, M., Vartiainen, P., Kiviranta, H. & Pekkanen, J. 2004. Risk–benefit analysis of eating farmed salmon. *Science*, 305(5683):476–477.

USEPA 2003. (cfpub.epa.gov/ncea/cfm/recordisplay.cfm?deid=87843)

USEPA 2005. Clean Air Mercury Rule (www.epa.gov/CAMR/).

USEPA, USFDA 2004. *What you need to know about mercury in fish and shellfish. Advice for women who might become pregnant, nursing mothers, young children.* United States Environmental Protection Agency and United States Food and Drug Administration (water.epa.gov/scitech/swguidance/fishshellfish/outreach/upload/2004_05_24_fish_MethylmercuryBrochure.pdf).

USFDA 2009. *Report of quantitative risk and benefit assessment of consumption of commercial fish, focusing on fetal neurodevelopment effects (measured by verbal development in children) and on coronary heart disease and stroke in the general population.* Draft report. United States Department of Health and Human Services, Food and Drug Administration (www.fda.gov/Food/FoodSafety/Product-SpecificInformation/Seafood/FoodbornePathogensContaminants/Methylmercury/ucm088758.htm).

Valera, B., Dewailly, E. & Poirier, P. 2009. Environmental mercury exposure and blood pressure among Nunavik Inuit adults. *Hypertension*, 54:981–986.

Vartiainen, T,, Jantunen, M., Miettinen, I., Nevalainen, A., Tuomisto, J. & Vilukselaan, M. 2006. Finland National Public Health Institute, Department of Environmental Health, Background Material for the International Evaluation
(www.ktl.fi/attachments/suomi/julkaisut/julkaisusarja_b/2006/2006b12.pdf).

Verbeke, W., Sioen, I., Pieniak, Z., Van Camp, J. & De Henauw, S. 2005. Consumer perception versus scientific evidence about health benefits and safety risks from fish consumption. *Public Health and Nutrition*, 8(4):422–429.

Verger, P., Houdart, S., Marette, S., Roosen, J. & Blanchemanche, S. 2007. Impact of a risk–benefit advisory on fish consumption and dietary exposure to methylmercury in France. *Regulatory Toxicology and Pharmacology*, 48(3):259–269.

Verger, P., Khalfi, N., Roy, C., Blanchemanche, S., Marette, S. & Roosen, J. 2008. Balancing the risk of dioxins and polychlorinated biphenyls (PCBs) and the benefit of long-chain polyunsaturated fatty acids of the n-3 variety for French fish consumers in western coastal areas. *Food Additives and Contaminants*, 25(6):765–771.

Virtanen, J.K., Voutilainen, S., Rissanen, T.H., Mursu, J., Tuomainen, T.P. & Korhonen, M.J. 2005. Mercury, fish oils, and risk of acute coronary events and cardiovascular disease, coronary heart disease, and all-cause mortality in men in eastern Finland. *Arteriosclerosis, Thrombosis, and Vascular Biology*, 25:228–233.

Wang, C.C., Harris, W.S., Chung, M., Lichtenstein, A.H., Balk, E.M., Kupelnick, B., Jordan, H.S. & Lau, J. 2006. n-3 fatty acids from fish or fish-oil supplements, but not alpha-linolenic acid, benefit cardiovascular disease outcomes in primary- and secondary-prevention studies: a systematic review. *American Journal of Clinical Nutrition*, 84(1):5–17.

Watzl, B., Gelencsér, E., Hoekstra, J.,Kulling, S.,Lydeking-Olsen, E. ,Rowland, I., Schilter, B., van Klaveren, J. & Chiodini, A. 2011. Application of the BRAFO-tiered approach for benefit–risk assessment to case studies on natural foods. *Food and Chemical Toxicology* [Epub ahead of print].

Weihe, P., Grandjean, P. & Jørgensen, P.J. 2005. Application of hair-mercury analysis to determine the impact of a seafood advisory. *Environmental Research*, 97(2):200–207.

WHO 1976. *Mercury*. Geneva, World Health Organization, 132 pp.(Environmental Health Criteria 1).

WHO 1998. Assessment of the health risks of dioxins: re-evaluation of the tolerable daily intake (TDI). *Executive Summary of the WHO Consultation*, May 25-29 1998, Geneva.

WHO 2000. *Assessment of the health risk of dioxins: Re-evaluation of the tolerable daily intake (TDI). WHO Consultation, Geneva, 25-29 May 1998*. Geneva, World Health Organization (www.who.int/ipcs/publications/en/exe-sum-final.pdf).

Wiseman, C.L.S. & Gobas, F. 2002. Balancing risks in the management of contaminated First Nations fisheries. *International Journal of Environmental Health Research*, 12(4):331–342.

Wong, E.Y., Ponce, R.A., Farrow, S., Bartell, S.M., Lee, R.C. & Faustman, E.M. 2003. Comparative risk and policy analysis in environmental health. *Risk Analysis*, 23(6):1337–1349.

World Cancer Research Fund, American Institute for Cancer Research 2007. *Food, nutrition, physical activity, and the prevention of cancer: a global perspective*, 2nd ed. Washington, DC, American Institute for Cancer Research.

Yokoyama, M., Origasu, H., Matsuzaki, M., Matsuzawa, Y., Saito, Y., Ishikawa, Y., Oikawa, S., Sasaki, J., Hishida, H., Itakura, H.,, Kita, T., Kitabatake, A., Nakaya, N., Sakata, T., Shimada, K. & Shirato, K. 2005. *Effects of eicosapentaenoic acid (EPA) on major cardiovascular events in hypercholesterolemic patients: the Japan EPA Lipid Intervention Study (JELIS)*. Presented at the American Heart Association Scientific Sessions, Late Breaking Clinical Trials II, 17 November 2005, Dallas, TX.

Yoshizawa, K., Rimm, E.B., Morris, J.S., Spate, V.L., Hsieh, C.C. & Spiegelman, D. 2002. Mercury and the risk of coronary heart disease in men. *New England Journal of Medicine*, 347:1755–1760.

Yuan, J.M., Ross, R.K., Gao, Y.T. & Yu, M.C. 2001. Fish and shellfish consumption in relation to death from myocardial infarction among men in Shanghai, China. *American Journal of Epidemiology*, 154:809–816.

APPENDIX A
ARITHMETIC MEAN CONTENT OF TOTAL FAT, EPA PLUS DHA, TOTAL MERCURY AND DIOXINS IN 103 SPECIES OF FISH

Common Name	Latin name	Arithmetic mean concentration				F/S/L
		Fat (g/100g)	EPA + DHA (mg/g)	Hg (µg/g)	Dioxins (pg TEQ/g)	
Alfonsino	*Beryx splendens*	9.00	11.40	0.71	0.51	F
Anchovy	*Engraulis encrasicolus*	3.39	17.00	0.04	2.47	F
Anglerfish	*Lophius piscatorius*	0.56	1.60	0.21	0.20	F
Bass, freshwater	*Micropterus* spp.	—	7.63	0.32	—	F
Bass, saltwater	*Morone saxatilis*	—	9.67	0.30	—	F
Bluefish	*Pomatomus saltatrix*	—	9.88	0.34	8.97	F
Butterfish	*Peprilus triacanthus*	—	1.90	0.06		F
Carp	*Cyprinus* spp.	—	4.51	0.20	—	F
Catfish	*Ictalurus* spp.	—	2.52	0.07	0.83	F
Catshark	*Scyliorhinus canicula, Scyliorhinus stellaris*	1.00	1.80	0.25	0.10	F
Clams	*Mercenaria spp*	—	1.77	0.02	0.11	S
Cockle	*Cerastoderma edule*	0.70	0.82	0.02	0.18	S
Cod, Atlantic (liver)	*Gadus morhua*	60.50	174.00	0.02	22.80	L
Cod, Atlantic (fillet)	*Gadus morhua*	0.81	2.10	0.09	0.11	F
Cod, Pacific	*Gadus macrocephalus*	0.20	1.00	0.09	0.035	F
Crab (brown meat)	*Cancer pagurus*	9.27	15.80	0.08	3.60	S
Crab (claw)	*Cancer pagurus*	1.01	7.00	0.12	3.33	S
Crab, spider	*Maja* spp.	6.90	8.31	0.03	5.58	S
Crawfish	*Procambarus clarkii*	—	1.64	0.03	0.15	S
Croaker, Atlantic	*Micropogonias undulatus*	—	2.02	0.07	—	F
Croaker, Pacific	*Genyonemus lineatus*	—	—	0.30	0.11	F
Cuttlefish	*Sepia officinalis*	1.66	2.25	0.04	0.16	S
Dab	*Limanda limanda, Microstomus kitt*	1.23	2.14	0.11	0.55	F
Eel	*Anguilla* spp.	26.90	18.90	0.20	49.81	F
Flatfish	*Hippoglossoides platessoides*	1.10	3.66	0.06	0.15	F
Goatfish	*Mullus barbattus, Mullus surmuletus*	5.90	10.17	0.12	2.61	F
Grenadier	*Coryphaenoides rupestris*	0.70	1.20	0.11	0.17	F
Grouper	*Epinephelus* spp.	—	2.48	0.46	—	F

Common Name	Latin name	Arithmetic mean concentration				F/S/L
		Fat (g/100g)	EPA + DHA (mg/g)	Hg (µg/g)	Dioxins (pg TEQ/g)	
Gurnard	*Trigla lucerna, Eutrigla gurnardus, Aspitrigla cuculus*	1.30	0.46	0.18	1.60	F
Haddock	*Melanogrammus aeglefinus*	0.54	1.70	0.09	0.13	F
Hake	*Merluccius* spp.	1.10	1.51	0.15	0.45	F
Halibut, Atlantic (farmed)	*Hippoglossus hippoglossus*	10.12	12.70	0.14	2.65	F
Halibut, Greenland	*Reinhardtius hippoglossoides*	11.70	10.50	0.23	3.70	F
Herring	*Clupea harengus*	12.60	19.40	0.04	3.84	F
Hoki	*Macruronus novaezelandiae*			0.19		F
John Dory	*Zeus faber*	1.00	3.40	0.08	0.50	F
Ling	*Molva* spp.	0.83	1.65	0.22	0.12	F
Lingcod and scorpionfish	*Ophiodon elongates* and *Scorpaenidae*	—	2.63	0.29	—	F
Lobster	*Hommarus* spp.	1.90	2.20	0.26	0.88	S
Lobster, American	*Hommarus americanus*	—	0.84	0.22	—	S
Lobster, Norway	*Nephrops norvegicus*	1.00	5.40	0.19	—	S
Lobsters, spiny	*Palinurus* spp.	—	4.80	0.12	—	S
Mackerel	*Scomber scombrus*	19.66	32.30	0.05	1.66	F
Mackerel, horse	*Trachurus trachurus*	15.80	14.50	0.11	1.10	F
Mackerel, king	*Scomberomorus cavalla*	—	4.01	0.73	—	F
Mackerel, Pacific	*Scomber japonicus*	12.10	20.84	0.11	1.30	F
Mackerel, Spanish	*Scomberomorus maculatus*	—	12.46	0.37	—	F
Marlin	*Makaira* spp.	0.20	0.30	0.78	0.02	F
Monkfish	*Lophius piscatorius*	—	—	0.20	—	F
Mussels	*Mytilus edulis*	1.90	3.30	0.04	0.63	S
Nile perch	*Lates niloticus*	1.63	2.50	0.12	—	F
Orange roughy	*Hoplostethus atlanticus*	—	0.31	0.58	0.40	F
Oysters	*Ostrea edulis*	1.46	0.90	0.01	0.90	S
Perch, freshwater	*Perca fluviatilis*	—	3.24	0.16	—	F
Perch, ocean and mullet	*Helicolenus percoides* and *Mullus* spp.	—	3.51	0.04	0.25	F
Periwinkle	*Littorina littorea*	3.10	2.86	0.01	0.15	S
Pike	*Esox lucius*	—	2.68	0.06	—	F
Plaice, European	*Pleuronectes platessa*	0.90	1.50	0.06	0.83	F
Pollock	*Pollachius pollachius*	0.63	2.50	0.05	0.21	F

Common Name	Latin name	Arithmetic mean concentration				F/S/L
		Fat (g/100g)	EPA + DHA (mg/g)	Hg (µg/g)	Dioxins (pg TEQ/g)	
Pout	*Trisopterus* spp.	0.50	0.66	0.15	0.23	F
Rainbow trout (farmed)	*Oncorhynchus mykiss*	11.30	19.40	0.05	1.02	F
Redfish	*Sebastes* spp.	4.30	8.30	0.05	0.48	F
Sablefish	*Anoplopoma fimbria*	—	18.12	0.27	—	F
Saithe (liver)	*Pollachius virens*	75.00	145.00	0.04	12.80	L
Saithe (fillet)	*Pollachius virens*	1.63	2.82	0.04	0.12	F
Salmon, Atlantic (wild)	*Salmo salar*	7.70	13.00	0.07	1.36	F
Salmon, Atlantic (farmed)	*Salmo salar*	12.60	21.30	0.05	1.63	F
Salmon, Pacific (wild)	*Oncorhynchus* spp.	7.80	11.60	0.04	0.25	F
Sardines	*Sardina pilchardus*	8.60	20.40	0.04	6.60	F
Scallops	*Pecten maximus*	1.17	2.10	0.02	0.64	S
Scampi	*Penaeus* spp.	1.15	2.60	0.07	0.14	S
Scorpion fish	*Scorpaena* spp.	4.00	6.28	0.17	2.20	F
Seabass	*Dicentrarchus labrax, D. punctatus*	4.80	9.74	0.14	3.86	F
Seabream	*Sparus aurata*	7.60	12.71	0.11	2.01	F
Sea urchin	*Strongylocentrus droebachiensis*	1.40	1.04	0.01	0.27	S
Shark	*Selachimorpha* spp.	—	3.70	0.80	0.09	F
Shrimp/prawn	*Pandalus borealis*	1.55	3.10	0.05	0.72	S
Skate/ray	*Raja* spp.	0.93	2.80	0.14	0.15	F
Smelt	*Osmerus eperlanus*	—	8.89	0.09	—	F
Snapper, porgy and sheepshead	*Lutijanus* spp.	—	2.56	0.14	—	F
Sole	*Solea* spp.	0.88	1.30	0.09	0.21	F
Sprat	*Sprattus sprattus*	10.98	19.40	0.04	4.96	F
Squid	*Loligo* spp.	1.33	3.50	0.10	0.87	S
Sweetfish	*Plecoglossus altivelis*	2.40	6.10	0.03	0.19	F
Swimcrab	*Liocarcinus corrugatus*	6.10	9.23	0.07	18.59	S
Swordfish	*Xiphias gladius*	8.00	6.80	1.05	0.92	F
Tilapia	*Tilapia* spp.	3.30	1.90	0.02	0.21	F
Tilefish, Atlantic	*Lopholatilus chamaeleonticeps*	—	9.05	0.11	—	F
Tilefish, gulf	*Caulolatilus microps*	—	—	1.45	—	F

		Arithmetic mean concentration				
Common Name	Latin name	Fat (g/100g)	EPA + DHA (mg/g)	Hg (µg/g)	Dioxins (pg TEQ/g)	F/S/L
Tuna	*Thunnus* spp.	3.88	7.70	0.49	1.91	F
Tuna, albacore	*Thunnus alalunga*	0.70	4.70	0.42	0.25	F
Tuna, Atlantic bluefin	*Thunnus thynnus*	—	—	0.69	—	F
Tuna, bigeye	*Thunnus obesus*	1.20	1.20	0.98	0.14	F
Tuna, Pacific bluefin	*Thunnus orientalis*	27.50	46.60	0.61	3.13	F
Tuna, skipjack	*Katsuwonus pelamis*	6.20	11.80	0.14	0.41	F
Tuna, yellowfin	*Thunnus albacares*	0.40	0.40	0.25	0.06	F
Turbot	*Rhombus maximus*	—	—	—	1.60	F
Tusk	*Brosme brosme*	0.90	1.80	0.15	0.13	F
Whelk	*Buccinum undatum*	1.60	1.59	0.05	0.68	S
Whiting	*Merlangius merlangus, Micromesistius poutassou*	0.54	1.20	0.18	0.21	F
Wild dogfish	*Squalus* spp.	—	—	—	2.20	F
Wolf fish	*Anarhichas lupus*	3.25	5.40	0.06	—	F

F = fish; S = shellfish; L = liver

[a] All concentrations are expressed per gram fresh weight.

APPENDIX B
MEETING PARTICIPANTS

Experts

Michael Bolger, Chief, Chemical Hazards Assessment Team, Center for Food Safety and Applied Nutrition, Food and Drug Administration, College Park, Maryland, USA

Laurie Chan, Professor, Community Health Sciences Program, University of Northern British Columbia, Prince George, British Columbia, Canada

Lucio Guido Costa, Professor, Department of Environmental and Occupational Health Sciences, School of Public Health and Community Medicine, University of Washington, Seattle, Washington, USA

Judy Cunningham, Principal Scientist, Food Composition, Evaluation and Modelling Section, Food Standards Australia New Zealand, Canberra, Australia

Elaine Faustman, Professor, School of Public Health and Community Medicine, University of Washington, Seattle, Washington, USA

Mark Feeley, Head, Food Contaminants Toxicology Evaluation, Chemical Health Hazard Assessment Division, Bureau of Chemical Safety, Health Canada, Ottawa, Ontario, Canada

Jeljer Hoekstra, Senior Researcher, Centre for Nutrition and Health, National Institute for Public Health and the Environment, Bilthoven, the Netherlands

Jean-Charles Leblanc, Head, Chemicals Exposure and Quantitative Risk Assessment, French Agency for Food, Environmental and Occupational Health Safety (ANSES), Maisons-Alfort, France

Anne-Katrine Lundeby-Haldorsen, Head, Research on Seafood Safety, National Institute of Nutrition and Seafood Research (NIFES), Nordnes, Bergen, Norway

Dariush Mozaffarian, Co-Director, Program in Cardiovascular Epidemiology, Harvard School of Public Health, Division of Cardiovascular Medicine, Harvard Medical School, Boston, Massachusetts, USA

Rachel Novotny, Professor, Human Nutrition, Food and Animal Science Department, College of Tropical Agriculture and Human Resources, University of Hawaii at Manoa, Honolulu, Hawaii, USA

Andrew J. Sinclair, Professor/Director, Metabolic Research Unit, School of Medicine, Deakin University, Waurn Ponds, Australia

Isabelle Sioen, Assistant Professor, Department of Public Health, Ghent University, Ghent, Belgium

J.J. (Sean) Strain, Director, Northern Ireland Centre for Food and Health, Centre for Molecular Biosciences, University of Ulster, Coleraine, Northern Ireland

Ricardo Uauy, Professor, Public Health Nutrition, London School of Hygiene and Tropical Medicine, University of London, London, England; Institute of Nutrition and Food Technology (INTA), Santiago, Chile

Yongning Wu, Professor, Department of Monitoring and Control for Contaminants, National Institute of Nutrition and Food Safety, Chinese Center for Disease Control and Prevention, Beijing, China

Michiaki Yamashita, Chief, Food Biotechnology Section, Biochemistry and Food Technology Division, National Research Institute of Fisheries Science, Fukuura, Kanazawa-ku Yokohama, Japan

Resource persons

Piotr Bykowski, Professor, Gdynia Maritime Academy, Gdynia, Poland

Clark D. Carrington, Pharmacologist, Office of Plants and Dairy Foods, Food and Drug Administration, College Park, Maryland, USA

Edel Oddny Elvevoll, Professor, Food Science, Department of Marine Biotechnology, Faculty of Biosciences, Fisheries and Economics, University of Tromsø, Tromsø, Norway

Food and Agriculture Organization of the United Nations (FAO)

Ichiro Nomura, Assistant Director-General, Fisheries and Aquaculture Department, FAO, Rome, Italy

Jean-Francois Pulvenis de Séligny, Fisheries and Aquaculture Policy and Economics Division, Fisheries and Aquaculture Department, FAO, Rome, Italy

Lahsen Ababouch, Fisheries and Aquaculture Products, Trade and Marketing Service, Fisheries and Aquaculture Policy and Economics Division, Fisheries and Aquaculture Department, FAO, Rome, Italy

Lourdes Costarrica, Nutrition and Consumer Protection Division, Agriculture and Consumer Protection Department, FAO, Rome, Italy

World Health Organization (WHO)

Hilde Kruse, Scientist, WHO Regional Office for Europe, European Centre for Environment and Health, Rome, Italy

FAO/WHO Secretariat

Grimur Valdimarsson, Special Advisor to Assistant Director-General, Fisheries and Aquaculture Department, FAO, Rome, Italy

Ruth Charrondiere, Nutrition and Consumer Protection Division, Agriculture and Consumer Protection Department, FAO, Rome, Italy

Kazuko Fukushima, Technical Officer, Department of Food Safety and Zoonoses, WHO, Geneva, Switzerland

Vittorio Fattori, Consultant, Nutrition and Consumer Protection Division, Agriculture and Consumer Protection Department, FAO, Rome, Italy

David James, Consultant, Fisheries and Aquaculture Products, Trade and Marketing Service, Fisheries and Aquaculture Policy and Economics Division, Fisheries and Aquaculture Department, FAO, Rome, Italy

Jogeir Toppe, Fishery Industry Officer, Fisheries and Aquaculture Products, Trade and Marketing Service, Fisheries and Aquaculture Policy and Economics Division, Fisheries and Aquaculture Department, FAO, Rome, Italy

Annika Wennberg, FAO Secretary to the Joint FAO/WHO Expert Committee on Food Additives, Nutrition and Consumer Protection Division, Agriculture and Consumer Protection Department, FAO, Rome, Italy